A Weight-Loss Guide for Menopause & Perimenopause

Hack Your Hormones for Weight-loss

PHYLLIS H. THOMPSON

Certified Personal Trainer
Integrative Nutritionist

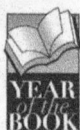

Year of the Book
135 Glen Avenue
Glen Rock, PA 17327

ISBN: 978-1-64649-383-8 (paperback)
ISBN: 978-1-64649-384-5 (ebook)

This book is not intended as a substitute for the medical advice of your physician. The reader should regularly consult a physician in matters relating to health before undertaking any exercise or diet change.

DEDICATION

To my late husband, Brett.
Your unconditional love helped me get here.
Thank you for always believing in me and
supporting all of my wild dreams...
And faking it when you didn't.
I love you and miss you dearly every day!

CONTENTS

*"Let food be thy medicine
and medicine be thy food."*

—Hippocrates

INTRODUCTION

For those of you who don't know me, I'm Phyllis Thompson... your favorite hormone-hacking coach for weight loss.

I am a certified integrative nutritionist and personal trainer. I am also an amateur fitness competitor. I've taken the stage three times and I'm going after my pro card.

I've been in fitness since 2014, though I didn't start to specialize in hormones until I personally started to feel the effects of perimenopause. Slimming down was tough, not to mention sleeping back then! Now, I help women age 35 and up to drop that unwanted weight by balancing their hormones.

When our hormone balance is off, the weight-loss technique of "calories in, calories out" doesn't always work. The simple math just isn't that simple.

Women dealing with a hormone imbalance face a myriad of struggles. Are you stuck with stubborn belly fat that just won't go away? Do you have hormonal symptoms that are the bane of your existence? Are you skipping the foods you genuinely enjoy so you can be in a calorie deficit... but the weight on the scale still isn't moving?

Trust me, I understand.

It's frustrating when your clothes don't fit the way they're supposed to. It can make you irritable on top of the mood swings you're already going through.

I used to love going out with my husband, but suddenly, I couldn't wear anything in my closet. Talk about a confidence buster. Girl, let me tell you about it! There were so many nights that I wanted us to go out, but... it's hard to be excited for a night on the town... especially in Atlanta, when you're worried about popping a zipper. That is often the case with most of us, isn't it? We gain just enough weight to make us want to hide indoors.

But what problem does that lead to?

Well, for starters, some of us get depressed. Right! We don't want to go out with our friends anymore.

We are apprehensive about undressing in front of our spouse... and forget being intimate.

We opt out of things we really want to do because we have nothing to wear... which is code for *nothing fits*.

And to add insult to injury, we stay home alone in front of the television... with a bag of chips or a whole container of ice cream. Now how are we gonna solve the belly bloat like that?

Let's shift gears for a bit. I invite you to think about how your life would change if you could actually lose weight and feel better. If you could follow a sustainable, effective, and easy plan, how would that change your life?

What are some of the things you would do differently after that?

> *How would your life change if you could finally reach your weight-loss goal?*

Once I lost the weight, I started to travel again and finally wore that bikini I had been eyeing for two years. Now I go out all the time. More importantly, I enjoy the process of getting ready. Remember those days as a young woman? We would spend hours on hair, makeup, and picking the perfect outfit to saunter out the door hours later, looking and feeling like a badass... with our confidence soaring. Losing the weight definitely brought back my confidence. And it all started with this hormone-hacking program.

This program is for you if you want to get rid of your belly bloat, unwanted weight, and those pesky symptoms, but don't know where to start. Or you've tried losing weight in the past, but either gained it all back or didn't have the success you wanted. Either way, I am here to tell you, it's likely not you;

it's usually your hormones that are keeping you from being great.

Hormones are the chemical messengers of our endocrine system, vital in controlling various bodily functions. But guess what? We have the power to influence how our hormones behave.

So much is within our control, but no one tells us that... especially not our doctors. And so many of them aren't teaching us preventative options because then they can't prescribe expensive medications or hormone therapies.

Side note: One of my clients told me: "Every time my doctor prescribes a medication, he's guaranteed to have to see me in three months." I will leave that there for you to do with what you will. In their defense, the professors didn't spend much study time on preventative natural remedies in medical school.

It's time for us to take back control of our bodies and put an end to accepting "your results are normal" from healthcare professionals. You can bio-hack your hormones and put those messengers to work for you!

In this book you'll discover how to balance your hormones so you speed up your metabolism... naturally. There are no magic potions, and no quick fixes. You won't have to rely on expensive hormone therapies that nobody knows for sure what the long-term effects are. We will do it holistically, with foods that work for us and not against us.

We will also uncover hidden weight-loss triggers that work while you sleep. And stress? Oh yeah. We will talk about stress relief that creates sustainable results for you. You've heard it before, and even though you probably can't wrap your head around it, stress can literally make you fat on a cellular level.

Sometimes, I can look at a woman and see it's all stress in her belly. If she could just get that under control, she could finally turn all her action into inches lost.

Now I want you to know that it's not your fault that you haven't been able to reach your goal thus far. It's possible that no one ever showed you the right way. What most people are doing just isn't helpful for you or your body.

Listen, our bodies are way different than when we were in our 20s. I'm 48 years old now and nothing that I used to do in my 20s works anymore. Until now, a puzzle piece was missing, and it could just be your hormones. But that all ends today.

A Vision for You

I want you to visualize something for me. I want you to imagine that you're no longer dealing with extra weight issues. The belly bloat is gone. You're in great shape. You feel good. You have more energy. You're not dealing with brain fog, low libido, hot flashes, night sweats, irritability, or mood swings any longer. You've reached your goal.

Close your eyes and mentally picture how you look and feel.

When you reopen your eyes, describe everything about that image to yourself. What were you wearing? Is there an outfit that signifies your success?

Who are you with? Maybe your spouse? Your sisters? Maybe your kids? Maybe your beau?

And how do you feel? That's the most important part. Do you have more energy? Do you feel good in your own skin? Are you clear-headed? Are you at peace with your body?

Now take a second and write that vision down... that is your goal!

Let me tell you about my client Heather, who dropped so much inflammation and bloat in her body that she can now wear her wedding rings again. There was a time when she couldn't—for two whole years. Talk about a blow to the ego! Once we got her hormones in check, all that inflammation disappeared. Her blood pressure dropped, and her doctor was able to reduce her medications. She even started hiking again. This was all done naturally with hormone-balancing nutrition and lifestyle change.

Think again about that mental picture of yourself after you've reached your goal. Like Heather, you'll eat delicious foods that energize you without giving up everything you love... because we all know, deprivation doesn't work. You'll start noticing your skin glowing and loving how you look and feel again. And you'll love the shape your body is taking.

Do you see that you can do it?

When I was overweight I didn't believe I could do it either. I have old pictures of me from before, and most people don't think it's me. Well, I wish it wasn't. Actually, I take that back... I learned so much from being the woman in the "before" picture. I just wish I'd learned it sooner.

Not only was I overweight. I was tired. I was unhappy, and I hated my body. Something had to change.

But what's funny is that I thought I was cute the day I took that picture... until I saw it later. I couldn't believe my eyes. I was saddened by how big I'd allowed myself to get. But the breakthrough came probably two years later. When I saw that picture again, I said, "Is that what I looked like?"

I was so tired of being embarrassed about my body. I was tired of hiding it from my husband. I was tired of not loving the image staring back at me in the mirror. More importantly, I was tired of not feeling good.

Years later this photo resurfaced. I couldn't get rid of this thing. We were at the Cheesecake Factory in Atlanta, waiting to be seated. My son's arm was wrapped around me and my husband decided to take a picture. Let me give you some context on what I looked like: This was back when I would drink myself to sleep every night... Well, not every night. Sometimes my body was so sick after multiple nights of heavy drinking that a couple of nights a week, I couldn't get the alcohol down, but not for lack of trying. And that's the unfortunate part.

> *I can't sit by and watch another woman go through what I endured.*

During the day, I was usually so hungover and in so much pain that I used food to get me through until I could drink again at night. Fried chicken, baked macaroni and cheese, and desserts... my comfort foods were heavy and fattening. Unbeknownst to me, I was also destroying my endocrine system and jacking up my hormones. I wouldn't find this out for a bit longer.

There were many photographs during my kids' childhood where I would later cut myself out of the images. Most of the time, though, I wouldn't let anyone take a picture of me. I couldn't look at the damage I'd done. Does that sound familiar?

So what turned things around for me? And more importantly, how can I turn things around for you?

Today is Your Someday

My *mess* became my *message.* I can't sit by and watch another woman go through what I endured. If you've been saying, "Someday I'm going to finally figure out how to lose that weight," then get ready. Today, you'll discover how to get your metabolism going, how to lose the belly bloat, shed that weight, and start living symptom-free... even if those hormones are a hot mess express right now.

The big elephant is still in the room though. I hear you. You don't want to give up all the foods you love. And you don't want to skip the holidays. Never mind wondering, "What if it doesn't work?" or "What if I can't stick to it?"

Don't worry! I will show you how to eat the foods you love in the right way. You won't have to give up bread, and we don't skip the holidays around here. Instead, you'll learn to enjoy every day the right way, so you never feel deprived, and so you stay on track with your goals.

Right now, you are on the cusp of making a lifestyle change. The first step was buying this book. Be proud of yourself for that... that was a boss move.

Unfortunately, that was the easy part. Right about now is usually when the fear sets in. The brain is designed to protect us, so it will come up with all sorts of reasons why you can't do this.

Maybe you're thinking, *"I won't succeed,"* or *"I'm not good enough."* Perhaps your worry is that the success won't last.

You're here to learn how to balance your hormones, lose weight, and sustain your long-term goals. These tips will become

You are on the cusp of making a lifestyle change.

such a habit that you won't even have to think about them later. It just takes practice and being shown the right way.

Failure is a real fear, and we all feel it when we face something new. But you won't have to worry about failure because I'm giving you all the tools to help you be successful.

Maybe you're worried you won't see results. This worry often happens to people who have tried something in the past and didn't get the expected outcome.

What if I told you I could hand you a solution designed for you to wipe away all of those fears and doubts? Failure is not an option. Instead you can have confidence that you will succeed...

Would you be in? I want to replace all those fears with your trust in the process... from wherever you're getting started... all the way to the finish line of your goals.

Plus it's simple to follow... so let's get started...

Write It Down for Success

I want you to find a piece of paper (preferably the one I had you write your vision on) and a pen. Why, you ask? Because true change requires some work... so let's get to work, shall we? Besides, a study by Harvard University says we are five times more likely to achieve our goals when we write them down. So now is your moment to increase the odds for yourself in a quick and easy way.

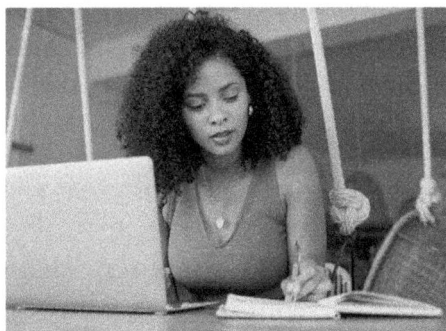

Write on that piece of paper, *"I'm ready to lose weight! I'm ready to feel confident in my own skin! I'm ready for permanent change."*

You can go a step further and set a date... make it realistic.

Time to Hack Those Hormones

So how are we going to get your hormones in check? It starts with foods that work for you and not against you. Then we'll hack the stress that's been weighing you down so you can finally lose that belly fat.

After that, you'll get the tools to hack your hormones through your gut (yeah, that's a real thing, and they are connected) to keep you healthy. Most of what ails us starts in the gut, and often when our hormones are out of balance, it's the foods we are eating that are making us sick—a vicious cycle.

I've also designed a fitness program you can use to get started. There's never any need to spend hours at the gym seven days a week. That just stresses your body out and makes it even harder for you to lose weight.

Next, I'm sharing my best hormone weight-loss suggested meal plans and recipes to boost your metabolism and alleviate symptoms. That way, you enjoy your most significant breakthrough of all. These take out all the guesswork at mealtime, so you don't have to worry about what to eat.

Even better, I will uncover the hidden weight-loss triggers that work while you sleep. You'll know exactly what your body needs to burn fat and stay balanced. And you'll learn how to sustain that.

Because I know you want to make the best-informed decisions for your health, I've also interviewed a functional medical doctor who shares her insider tips on hormones and weight loss.

Bonuses!

You'll get the hormone-balancing foods cheat sheet, so you know at a glance what foods will keep you balanced or imbalanced, and why. You want sustained progress, right? When you know what foods work for you, and what foods sabotage you, it's easier to make better choices.

There's also a cheat sheet for the nutrients your body needs at this stage of life because, as I said earlier, it's no longer as simple as just calories in and calories out. Specific nutrients give your body what it needs to make the hormones you're lacking, metabolize those you have in excess, and support other systems and processes so you function optimally. These foods help keep your energy up and help you sleep better.

Finally, you get the daily weight-loss checklist, which will serve as your blueprint. It will help you bring it all together with a few things to check off daily to help you reach and sustain your desired results and keep you in balance.

Are you ready to get started? Let's jump right in!

Chapter 1

Hack Your Hormones with Food

Most women over the age of 35 struggle with weight gain, and despite their efforts, find it challenging to lose weight... and not for lack of trying. I mean, most of us are giving an all-out effort here. But our hormones are holding us back, and they don't know that in most cases.

You could be eating right and doing all the exercises, but still just spinning your wheels. Knowing what to do so that your weight loss efforts are actually more effective will make a *huge* and immediate difference for you.

So, how will we dump that unwanted weight and speed up your metabolism naturally with foods that work for you, not against you?

One of the easiest ways to maintain hormonal balance is through diet, and when I use the word diet, I mean your daily nutrition. You're probably wondering, "Well, what foods *can* I eat then?" My question to you is, "Are you ready?" Let's go!

Hormone Nourishing Foods

So many delicious food choices will help balance your hormones naturally.

First up, avocado... it's super healthy. It's actually a fruit, if you didn't know that. It has sufficient beta-sitosterol (a plant compound) that can positively affect cholesterol levels in the blood. Cholesterol is what our body uses to make our hormones.

Avocados also help level out your cortisol, the stress hormone, which inadvertently makes losing weight a battle. The more stressed you are, the more cortisol attaches to the adipose tissue (the fat cells) in your belly, which makes it even harder to lose belly fat. Avocado can help level that out. Hecks yeah! How about some avocado toast for breakfast :)

These delicious foods help balance your hormones naturally.

Next up are Brazil nuts which are densely loaded with selenium and serve as an antioxidant in the body. There's also selenium in eggs. Selenium is an essential mineral that is particularly crucial for regulating thyroid function. Our thyroid is a mighty little guy that does many things, including regulating our metabolism. Our metabolism is the rate at which our body burns food... i.e., energy. So if you deal with thyroid issues, I would discuss that with your doctor and consider adding it to your routine.

Then there is calcium, which helps prevent PMS. Broccoli is a vegetable that is rich in calcium.

I will pause right here and talk about calcium relating to milk. This is one of my soapbox issues. Non-organic cow's milk is so inflammatory. It's one of the worst things we can consume when we're over 35. Instead, you can get calcium from leafy greens and other green vegetables—like broccoli. Broccoli is also known to help maintain healthy estrogen levels in the body.

When your estrogen and progesterone are out of balance, it throws everything off.

There are things called Xeno estrogens, which act like estrogen but are not. They attach to the estrogen receptors in your body, making you estrogen-dominant. Estrogen dominance can present as belly fat, mood swings, breast tenderness, and a whole host of other issues. Broccoli is an easy way to care for your calcium needs while also helping prevent estrogen dominance and PMS.

Broccoli also contains a compound called Diindolylmethane (DIM for short). DIM has been shown to enhance estrogen metabolism and aids in the elimination of excess estrogens from your body.

Foods rich in DIM (including cruciferous veggies like broccoli, cauliflower, and cabbage) can be beneficial for minimizing hot flashes, night sweats, mood swings and joint pain. Umm!! You had me at hot flashes... put some of that on my plate.

Flax seeds are another must-have. They are a significant supplier of phytoestrogens (plant estrogens), including ligands, which work to prevent certain types of cancers. These super seeds contain omega-3 fatty acids, which have anti-inflammatory properties. These anti-inflammatory properties also help with joint pain. Flax seeds are also known for balancing the progesterone and estrogen ratio in the body. Flax seeds are a great addition to oatmeal or smoothies.

Iodine-rich foods are another important addition for the production of thyroid hormones. Now that most of us have stopped using iodized table salt, it's important to intentionally consume iodine-rich foods. Remember our thyroid regulates our metabolism. Often the shift in hormones at this stage can trigger a thyroid disorder... so consider being proactive here and take some preventative measures.

Women with thyroid disorders should increase their intake of seafood, sea vegetables, and pasture-raised eggs to prevent an iodine deficiency. It is essential to discuss testing your iodine levels with your doctor before you increase consumption of these foods for this purpose.

You can also buy dried seaweed in the grocery store, and now they come in flavors like sea salt, wasabi, and chili lime... so have fun with it. Those are so easy to add to your nutrition because all you have to do is grab a couple of slices and put them into your mouth... so easy!

Eggs are also super easy, but because they have a lot of cholesterol, I suggest using two whole eggs plus egg whites as a filler, so you don't get the extra fat from the yolks—because that's where the majority of the fat is.

Seafood is simple to get in some parts of the country. Fish and shellfish are low in saturated fat and contain high-quality protein, omega-3 fatty acids, and other essential nutrients. A well-balanced diet that includes a variety of seafood can contribute to heart health. Opt for wild-caught when you can, as farm-raised sea proteins aren't always fed the best food.

You already know the importance of leafy greens for your health. But let's expand on that in the context of hormone health. Green vegetables, such as spinach and kale, are rich in essential nutrients which contribute to balancing hormones in the body.

These veggies are packed with antioxidants. Increasing consumption of these powerhouse veggies can also combat inflammation, a fundamental factor in many health problems, including the joint pain we discussed earlier. They also help fight against osteoporosis, which is a major concern in the menopause years.

Side note: Weight-bearing exercise is another simple and great way to prevent osteoporosis.

Now, let's get back to leafy greens. They also contain magnesium, which can help manage stress by regulating the production of stress hormones our bodies produce.

In addition to improving cortisol levels, these vegetables are also a great source of iron, which is required for normal thyroid functioning.

Moreover, these vegetables can also help you get your estrogen back in balance... think about getting rid of mood swings and excess belly fat when we talk about estrogen balance.

They're also perfect for getting nice, bulky, low-calorie foods that are nutrient-dense into our bodies.

Vegetables like spinach, kale, and chard do even more for our hormones. The downside is that spinach and kale tend to be at the top of the list of the worst offenders for pesticides, and heavy pesticides are endocrine disruptors. (An endocrine disruptor is any chemical that interferes with your body's hormone system.)

Don't splurge on "organic" for foods with thick skin—like bananas and navel oranges.

Buying organic is not the most budget friendly, but it will be much better for you than eating spinach laced with pesticides. Besides, the more we buy it, the lower the costs will be as the demand for organic produce rises. In the interim, shop at your local farmers' market, or look for mark-downs as organic produce gets close to its shelf date. Then take advantage of the savings when you can. Note that some fruits and veggies are not necessary to buy organic, Like for example, anything with thick skin—like bananas and navel oranges. The thicker skin makes it harder for pesticides to get into the fruit.

Next up... Pomegranates. I love pomegranates, and not just because they are ripe for picking in my birthday month. They are not only delicious, they are amazing. You may find them in grocery stores at other times of year, but they'll be sweetest in the fall... just like me... haha!!

Pomegranates are an excellent source of antioxidants. Eating this fruit can help with vaginal dryness, hot flashes, and night sweats, and some studies suggest it can improve libido. *Hello*, you had me at libido! Ummmm! Have I used that line already?

Eating pomegranate can also help with PMS, and it helps regulate monthly periods and promotes fertility in women.

Lastly, this fruit also supplies sufficient potassium and vitamin C levels necessary for thyroid function.

You can get pomegranate extract or juice when pomegranates are not in season. But it may have fillers or added sugars, depending on who makes it. Beware of added sugar! READ THE LABEL!!!

Client Spotlight time

Meet Apryl, a shining example of success. Despite her busy travel schedule for work, Apryl mastered the art of eating well on the go. She embraced my hormone-balancing recipes, significantly reduced her fast-food intake, and incorporated more fresh produce into her diet.

The result? An incredible 40-pound weight loss journey. Apryl's newfound vitality even allowed her to lead a mountain climbing adventure in Spain in her 50s, where she was moving faster than the younger women in the group.

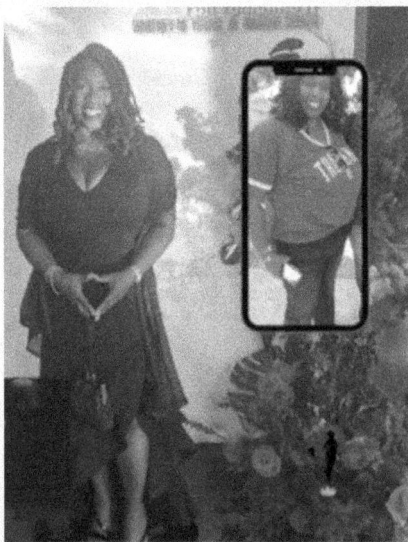

Talk about aging for longevity. Apryl also completed her first 5k while in our program. Apryl shares: "Before joining your hormone hacking program, the idea of eating to lose weight was baffling to me. I always thought to lose weight, I had to starve myself. I couldn't fathom not only eating, but eating delicious food, and still losing weight. This program illuminated the link between enjoying delicious, nutritious food and shedding pounds. Now, I find myself dining out less, cooking more at home, and surprisingly, becoming a regular fresh produce buyer. Who would have thought?"

During the course of our program, Apryl came out of her shell. She starting dating more, wearing more colorful clothes, and showing more skin. She realized the beautiful side-effect of taking care of herself is having more confidence.

Your Food Journal

Look again at the list of hormone-nourishing foods above and see which ones are already part of your weekly nutrition. Cross those off because you're already getting them. Pick 1 or 2 things you want to consume more regularly and add those in this week.

After two weeks of adding that one thing in, pick something different. It's essential to see how your body and your system respond to new foods. I recommend starting a journal where you keep notes about the food you eat and how it affects your mood, your body, and your symptoms.

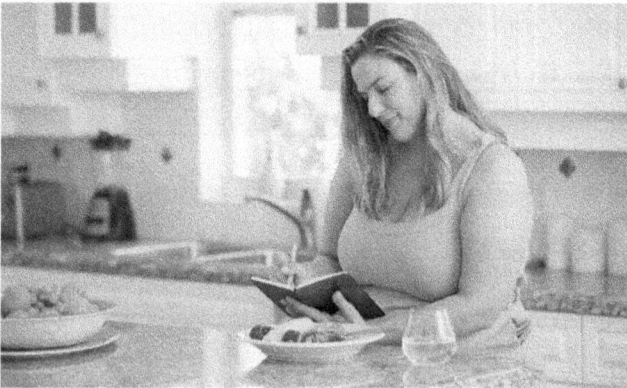

Whenever you note a food or ingredient that affects your body negatively, you don't want to keep that around. Take it out of your diet. Get it out of your house.

The reason to only introduce only one or two new foods at a time is that if you add too many at once, you won't know which one is causing the changes your body is experiencing, positive or negative.

Side note: You are provided with a checklist in your bonuses. Write down the 1 or 2 foods you will add on that sheet so you have a clear game plan when you are done reading this book.

That leads us into foods to avoid.

Foods to Avoid

Now what foods do you need to avoid? Those are pretty easy. They're the same ones that you should avoid for weight gain.

If you want to balance your hormones, lose weight, be healthy, and live symptom-free for longevity, then it's time to cut down on alcohol.

Alcohol spikes hot flashes, just like sugars—corn syrup, white sugar, and brown sugar—which are known for worsening hormone imbalance and increasing the chances of insulin resistance.

Alcohol spikes hot flashes.

Suppose you have been on a health and fitness or weight-loss journey before. In that case, I'm sure you've heard about insulin resistance, especially for those of us over a certain age. Sugar makes that worse. Avoiding processed sugars helps you to maintain hormonal balance while also assisting you in losing weight.

Some trainers believe there is not a difference between fruit sugars and alcohol sugars... but that is absolutely untrue. Your body knows the difference!

Fruit sugars and raw honey are natural. They contain enzymes that your body is equipped to break down and utilize.

Table sugar is processed sugar, as is corn syrup. Your body is not designed to break those things down.

Alcohol in your body is treated like processed sugar and it can spike hot flashes.

Sugar and alcohol can remain in your system for days, affecting your body long after the moment when you consume it.

For me, alcohol is no longer in my diet. I can still remember the horrible anxiety that came along with my drinking. I remember driving my kids one rainy day, and even though I hadn't been drinking that day, the alcohol still in my system from the day before caused me to have the worst anxiety attack. Scientifically I knew I wasn't dying; it was a panic attack. I had to repeat to myself over and over, "You have too much adrenaline going through your system right now. This is your body's response to it. You are NOT dying." Eventually the feeling went away.

Alcohol and sugar will both spike your anxiety.

Alcohol may not be so challenging to eliminate for some, and if it is, we might have a bigger problem. If you're a nightly drinker and you suffer from hot flashes, I strongly suggest you cut out the alcohol right away.

There's nothing wrong with having a drink a couple of times a month. But if alcohol is a part of your daily routine, and it's making you have hot flashes or night sweats, then you can make a different choice from a place of empowerment. You won't have to feel deprived. When you know the negative ways alcohol affects you, you can make the choice to not consume it, or to indulge in the spirits a bit less... because you want to feel better and enjoy life more.

Alcohol and sugar both spike anxiety, which can worsen as we are going through hormonal changes. One of my clients had experienced debilitating anxiety for *years*. We created a custom plan with a primary focus on her nutrition, and... legit... in five days, she reported back, "I don't wake up riddled with anxiety anymore." This was above and beyond her excitement over the weight she lost. She was just so happy to not have that debilitating anxiety.

Caffeine is another known offender, as it can also spike hot flashes and anxiety and disrupt your sleep. This includes coffee, soda, tea, and those energy drinks.

Reduce your caffeine intake GRADUALLY.

Caffeinated drinks can be really difficult to come off of because your body literally gets addicted. Caffeine withdrawal can be really challenging as well. It could lead to headaches, decreased motivation, and irritability. Nobody enjoys that. It can even be worse than the symptoms of not getting enough sleep.

As you try to reduce your caffeine intake, use a gradual approach. Remove one cup of coffee or other caffeinated drink from your diet daily. After a week, then remove one more.

Like caffeine, sugar is addictive and can be difficult to come off of as well. You will want to reduce it in the same way I mentioned above. Take away one sugar-filled item per day or every other day each week. Then, continue to reduce your sugar intake each week after that, and you will see the benefits.

A study published in the *British Journal of Sports Medicine* revealed that, in testing with rats, sugar is more addictive than opioid drugs like cocaine. Both sugar and cocaine addiction in rats (and humans) led to predictable behaviors that could be observed—bingeing, craving, tolerance, withdrawal, dependence, and reward.

In the new study, lab rats were given access to a set of levers eight times a day. One lever released cocaine, and the other released water laced with refined sugar. While both had been proven to be addictive in previous studies, the rats went back for the sugar when given a choice.

Imagine! Sugar is more addictive than a narcotic drug. And the more you put it into your body, the more it makes you want it.

One of the best ways to start to eliminate processed sugar is to temporarily increase your intake of fresh fruit in season. When it's in season, the fruit is at its sweetest. Try to get your fruit from a local farmers' market. Whenever you would usually eat something with refined sugar, have a piece of fresh fruit instead.

I also like putting lemon and cucumber slices in my water when coming off sugar. It naturally sweetens the water, and staying hydrated helps as well.

Replace processed sugars with fresh fruit at first.

Another thing to try during your break-up with sugar is eating more healthy fats, like avocado. I love a good avocado toast with organic grape tomatoes and pasture-raised eggs on gluten-free bread for breakfast. Couple that with some fresh seasonal fruit and you've got a breakfast that will energize and satisfy you and help you ditch the sluggish feeling often associated with sugar.

Coming off of sugar can be a process. It's not something you should try to accomplish overnight. Otherwise, you'll go spiraling back headfirst into a vat of ice cream because you are so tired of being miserable... or maybe that's just me...

Reducing your sugar intake also affects the dopamine levels in your brain. Dopamine is responsible for the feeling of pleasure. Because sugar affects the dopamine, if you try to cut out all sugar at once, that can be rough. It can even cause depression. Remove a little at a time and notice how your body responds. I can't stress that enough... that is where your empowerment comes from. We want to make choices from a place of power (knowing how we want to feel) and not a place of deprivation. Keep track of that in a journal or the checklist provided in your bonuses so you have a clear game plan, and then decide how you want to lower your sugar intake in the weeks ahead.

Empowerment, Not Deprivation

Hormone health really is in your hands, because only you are responsible for your food choices.

I firmly believe that when you're armed with knowledge about why to choose certain foods over others, it will come from a place of empowerment rather than deprivation.

You won't feel like you're being cheated out of anything.

When the conversation in your head changes from, "Oh, I can't have this food because I'm trying to lose weight," and shifts to, "I can have that if I want to, but I know that it's going to make me feel bad," that knowledge and education is empowering.

You no longer feel like you're being cheated out of anything. You're making decisions from a place of self-confidence rather than emotional resentment.

The most effective way to control your endocrine health, which controls your hormones, is by controlling your nutrition. The food you choose to eat is your first line of defense.

Let's talk about some of these hormones for a second.

Estrogen

One of those hormones that changes as you age is estrogen. Leading up to menopause (the perimenopause phase) estrogen can be all over the place and then it declines by 40 to 60 percent during menopause, just enough to make the monthly cycles stop. But what most women don't know is perimenopause and its symptoms can start up to 10 years before you go into menopause. For some women that is around age 35. The symptoms are pretty much the same for both stages, too, so getting ahead of it in perimenopause means by the time you get to menopause, it will be a much smoother transition.

The absence of your monthly cycle for 12 consecutive months is what signals true menopause.

The fluctuation of estrogen levels during both stages is, in part, responsible for those pesky symptoms like hot flashes, poor quality of sleep, and vaginal dryness.

Most of the body's estrogen is produced by the ovaries, which will stop during menopause. The drop in estrogen can also have a significant impact on your mood, making you feel anxious, depressed, and stressed.

Thankfully the adrenal glands—those triangular shaped glands that sit on top of the kidneys—are also responsible for making a small percentage of our estrogen and progesterone. So we must take care of those glands sooner rather than later.

Some women go through all of the symptoms of perimenopause and menopause with great difficulty and discomfort while others experience fewer and more subtle symptoms.

Your symptoms and their severity greatly depend on your individual and familial history. More often than not, what your mother experienced during menopause can tell you a lot about what's in store for you. Until now! I am going to show you how to thrive during these times.

In addition to the decrease in your estrogen levels, progesterone levels also decrease during menopause. Progesterone is our "keep calm" hormone… think reduced anxiety when we talk about progesterone. As mentioned before, the first step in feeling better and getting that hormonal weight off is eliminating foods known to disrupt hormonal balance, and the best time to start is in perimenopause. That so eloquently leads us to…

Foods to Avoid or Use Less Frequently:

- **Conventional dairy:** Because they are high in lactose and also filled with antibiotics and steroids, foods like cream cheese, ice cream, custard, and butter should be avoided.

- **Gluten:** Foods like white bread, beer, cakes, cookies, and cereal are high in gluten, which can derail your weight loss goals and impact gut health.

- **Refined sugar:** It's no surprise that candy, cakes, cookies, pie, ice cream, and doughnuts are high in refined sugar, but also avoid or cut down your intake of sweetened drinks including soft drinks, sports drinks, energy drinks, and juice drinks.

- **Industrialized cooking oils:** These seed oils are heated to extremely high temperatures, which cause oxidation of the fatty acids, creating by-products that harm your health. Avoid canola, corn, cottonseed, soy, sunflower, and grapeseed oils.

- **Coffee:** While caffeine can boost energy levels, it is also known to disrupt estrogen production and spike hot flashes. Look for Fairtrade and organic brands.

- **Alcohol:** Due to its effect on the liver, alcohol use is linked to impaired production of progesterone and an increased risk of breast cancer.

- **Processed foods:** Because they increase inflammation and stress the adrenal glands, avoid processed foods, including soy and dairy products.

- **Foods with chemicals:** Several canned and processed foods are tainted by toxic chemicals. Avoid items with palm oil, shortening, high-fructose corn syrup, food dyes, and MSG.

Produce Selection

How can you naturally support the balance of estrogen levels?

Remember, when selecting food, it's always best to go organic to avoid toxins like pesticides, fungicides, herbicides, and GMOs, which all can disrupt the endocrine system.

Each year, the Environmental Working Group creates the "Clean 15" and "Dirty Dozen" lists so you know which produce is essential to buy organic.

This Year's "Dirty Dozen" to AVOID

- Strawberries
- Spinach
- Kale, collard and mustard greens
- Peaches
- Pears
- Nectarines
- Apples
- Grapes
- Bell and hot peppers
- Cherries
- Blueberries
- Green beans

According to the Environmental Working Group's research, more than 90 percent of samples of strawberries, apples, cherries, spinach, nectarines, and grapes tested positive for residues of two or more pesticides.

A total of 210 pesticides were found on Dirty Dozen items. Of those, over 50 different pesticides were detected on every type of crop on this list, except cherries.

All of the produce on the Dirty Dozen had at least one sample with at least 13 different pesticides, and some had as many as 23.

This Year's "Clean Fifteen"

Foods with the lowest amounts of pesticide residues include:

1. Avocados
2. Sweet corn
3. Pineapple
4. Onions
5. Papaya
6. Sweet peas (frozen)
7. Asparagus
8. Honeydew melon
9. Kiwi
10. Cabbage
11. Mushrooms
12. Mangoes
13. Sweet Potatoes
14. Watermelon
15. Carrots

Almost 65 percent of Clean Fifteen fruit and vegetable samples had no detectable pesticide residues. Avocados and sweet corn were the cleanest produce noted.

Vitamins

Remember those adrenal glands I mentioned earlier... which also make small amounts of our sex hormones? During perimenopause and menopause it is vital to support those glands since they will be taking over for the ovaries when they retire. The sooner you start supporting them, the better.

Vitamin E plays an important role in supporting the adrenal glands. When the adrenal glands function properly, as your ovaries stop producing estrogen, these glands will continue producing and releasing some estrogen into the bloodstream. Research has also shown that vitamin E helps ease symptoms like night sweats and hot flashes.

My big rule of thumb is to supplement with real food first. If that isn't cutting it, discuss other forms of supplementation with your doctor beforehand to make sure you aren't getting too much of something and there aren't any drug interactions.

Natural food sources of vitamin E include sunflower seeds, avocados, almonds, Swiss chard, and butternut squash. But remember that when it comes to nuts and seeds, you want to consume them raw, as the roasting process breaks down some of their fatty acids and natural nutrients.

The B vitamins—especially vitamin B5—have several functions including the regulation and support of the adrenal glands. They play a role in synthesizing cholesterol, the precursor to all the hormones, including estrogen and progesterone.

B vitamins are also heavily involved in energy production and therefore help with memory, regulating your mood, and helping you think clearly.

Since "brain fog" is a very common symptom during this stage of life—when you have difficulty concentrating and feel forgetful—the B vitamins can help.

Vitamin B5 is naturally found in chicken, oats and other whole grains, eggs, beef, and potatoes.

We all know **vitamin C** is great for the immune system, but it also provides adrenal support. A diet rich in vitamin C makes sure they can function properly and keep the hormones balanced.

Vitamin C also protects against bone loss since it's an essential nutrient in the synthesis of collagen. Collagen is the protein in bones and connective tissue that keeps them durable and strong. Not to mention, collagen helps our skin look younger for longer.

Citrus fruits, like lemons and oranges, grapefruits, red peppers, and Brussels sprouts, all contain a high percentage of the daily recommended vitamin C intake.

Fun fact: One orange contains over 100 percent of the necessary vitamin C!

The Plant Benefit—bonuses to eating all these plants

Phytoestrogens are natural compounds found in plant foods that can weakly bind to the body's estrogen receptors and aid in the balance of estrogen levels. Though gentler, they closely resemble human estrogens in their chemical structure, with only 2 percent of the estrogenic activity of human estrogen.

While less potent, unlike human estrogens, they are freely available to the tissues. They can also act as a buffer if too much estrogen is in the body. This can help metabolize excess estrogen produced from chemicals in your skin care, home care, and environment, which enables you to stay balanced. These chemicals are the Xeno-estrogens (fake estrogens) I mentioned earlier. So load up on plants!

Your health is truly in your hands. You have more input than you think! But to make it easier, I have included a 28-day suggested hormone-balancing meal plan with all the recipes in this book. You have it all, including a shopping list for the grocery store. You can find it on page 113 at the back if you're ready to dive straight in!

Super Savvy Tip

Download your FREE copy of
my beautiful, full-color
4-week Meal Plan and Recipe Bundle:

hackyourhormonesforweightloss.com/bonuses

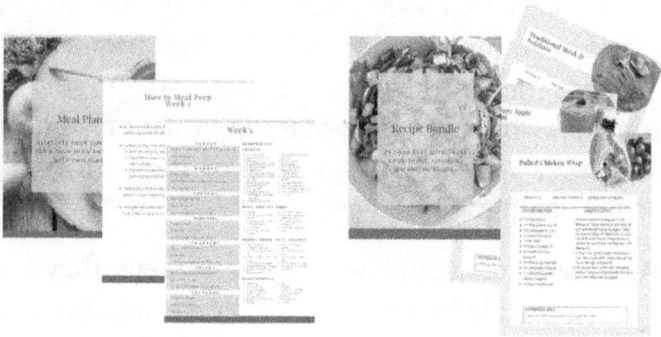

CHAPTER 2

Hack Your Stress

If your stress hormones are imbalanced, you may experience muscle weakness, salt cravings, low blood pressure, hypoglycemia, fatigue, anxiety, inability to sleep and even panic attacks. Sheesh!!

Cortisol, our stress hormone, flows through our body in a rhythm throughout the day. It's higher in the morning when we wake and should be lower at night to help us fall asleep. But when that system isn't functioning properly, it will be high when it should be low or low when it should be high. This can cause sleep disturbances and feelings of anxiety due to its activation of your body's fight or flight response.

High cortisol can also lower your progesterone, which again is our keep-calm hormone. This is yet another way cortisol increases feelings of anxiety, especially in the menopause years when progesterone starts to dip.

Your body's fight or flight response mobilizes the stored form of sugar (glycogen). It converts it to glucose so it's ready for use. Still, if you aren't truly going to use that energy to, say... run from a threat... your body will then store what cannot be converted back to glycogen as fat in the adipose tissue (fat cells).

Guess which part of the body has the most fat cells... You guessed it, our bellies. Good job, class.

In this way, stress hinders weight loss and can cause weight gain. Effectively handling stress and ensuring adequate quality sleep are essential for maintaining hormonal balance, particularly during this significant phase of life. In my program, we focus on

> *Stress not only hinders weight loss... it can cause weight gain.*

uncovering stress-relief techniques and sleep enhancement strategies that are uniquely suited to your individual needs.

Envision yourself waking up each morning feeling rejuvenated and eager to face the day's challenges. Our goal is to turn this vision into your daily reality.

Let me introduce you to Shanai, whom we affectionately referred to as "the sleepless workaholic."

This remarkable woman runs two thriving businesses, all while fulfilling her roles as a wife and mother. Her hectic lifestyle led to persistent anxiety and sleep disturbances. Our collaborative efforts uncovered a direct link between her weight gain and her body's stress response. Like we do with all our clients, we fine-tuned Shanai's nutrition. We introduced personalized lifestyle modifications that soothed her system, including recommendations for adaptogens like Rhodiola to help her body manage stress better. This reduced her anxiety, improved her sleep quality, and restored her vitality. The result? An incredible loss of over 40 inches and 30 pounds. Shanai joyfully shares that she feels like she's regained her mojo, a testament to the transformative power of our program.

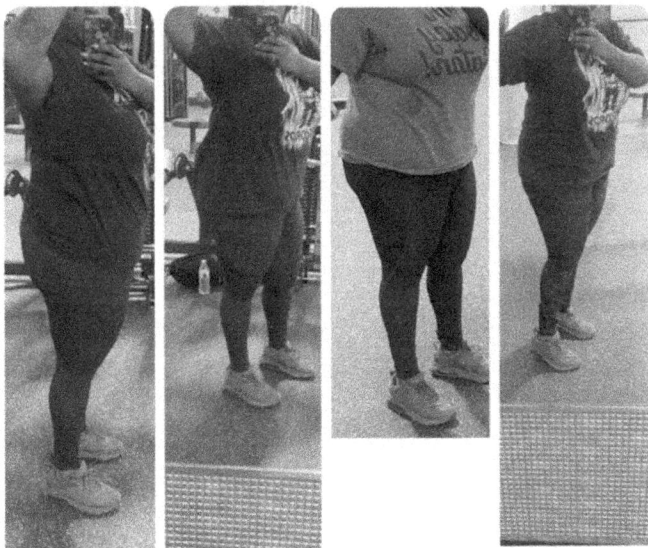

One of my favorite stress-relieving techniques I recommend to some of my clients is box breathing. It's used by Navy Seals to help them remain calm in stressful situations. If it's good enough for the Seals, it's good enough for us.

Box Breathing

Here how I recommend using it. The next time you find yourself in a stressful situation, whether it be rush-hour traffic, a screaming child, or a spouse you want to punch in the face... (just kidding... no hitting spouses) try this:

Step 1:

Slowly inhale through your nose for 4 seconds.

Step 2:

Hold at the top of the inhale for 4 seconds.

Step 3:

Slowly exhale through your mouth for 4 seconds.

Step 4:

Hold at the bottom of the exhale for 4 seconds.

Didn't that feel good?

Why Box Breathing Helps

- Lowers stress and anxiety by reducing cortisol levels, which is crucial for hormonal balance.

- Improves focus and concentration.

- Enhances sleep quality, aiding in overall well-being.

- Lowers blood pressure, proven to be beneficial for heart health.

Practice daily for 4 or 5 cycles for optimal results. Ideal for moments of high stress or before bedtime.

Meditation

Another technique I like to recommend is meditation. Meditation is a mind-body practice that enhances mental clarity, emotional calmness, and physical relaxation through techniques like mindfulness, breathing, and focused attention. There are countless research studies on its benefits, including but not limited to reduced inflammation, reduced stress, and improved sleep. Best of all, it has recently been proven that meditation can help prevent brain degenerative disorders. I'll take that benefit for two hundred, Alex...

Here's a little guide in case you are new to the practice.

Step 1: Find a Quiet Space

Choose a peaceful area where you won't be disturbed. This could be a corner of your room, office, a comfortable chair, or even a spot in your garden.

Step 2: Set a Timer

Start with short sessions, like 3-5 minutes, and gradually increase the duration as you get more comfortable.

Starting with shorter times also makes it fit easily into your daily routine.

Step 3: Get Comfortable

Sit or lie down in a comfortable position. Sit on a chair or lie on your back.

Step 4: Focus on Your Breath

Close your eyes and bring your attention to your breathing. Breathe naturally, observing the sensation of your breath as it enters and leaves your body.

Step 5: Notice When Your Mind Wanders

Your mind will wander; it's natural. Gently acknowledge these thoughts and then return your focus to your breath. This is why it's called a practice... you get better with time, so show yourself some grace and be proud you are putting in the effort.

Step 6: Close Your Session

Gently open your eyes and take a moment to notice your environment and how your body feels.

Benefits of Meditation

- Transitioning smoothly back to your day, you carry the calmness and clarity you claimed in your meditation.

- Regular meditation can significantly lower stress and anxiety levels, which is crucial for hormonal balance during perimenopause and menopause.

- Improves sleep quality.

- Enhances mood and emotional wellbeing.

- Increases focus and mental clarity.

Better physical health. Regular practice can enhance cognitive function, helping to combat the "brain fog" often experienced during perimenopause and menopause.

Meditation enhances immune function, reduces blood pressure, and is vital for overall health during hormonal change.

If you need a little more guidance with meditation, I recommend the Calm app. You can use the free version, which has a relaxation and breathing meditation that takes you through a sequence set to calming background sounds like nature or soothing music. I have a former client, NeKe, who loves evening meditation before bed... she says it helps her sleep better. I prefer to meditate in the morning, during my quiet time, before I start my day. Play around with different times and find what feels good to you.

Yoga

I personally love a good hot yoga class. I walk out feeling zen, clear-headed, and focused. Often, yoga is referred to as a "moving meditation." They call it that because it combines physical movement with mindfulness and focused breathing, creating a meditative state through motion.

Yoga is highly beneficial for managing stress. Its gentle stretches and poses help release tension from the body. At the same time, deep breathing techniques promote relaxation and mental clarity, effectively reducing stress and anxiety.

The meditative aspect of yoga encourages mindfulness, which can help break the cycle of stress-related thoughts.

For those looking to start a yoga practice, beginning with basic poses like Child's Pose, Cat-Cow Stretch, and simple breathing exercises can be a great way to ease into a routine. Many online resources and apps offer beginner-friendly yoga sessions.

Joining a local class can provide guidance and a sense of community. Many yoga studios offer new student promotions. For example, Corepower Yoga (where I got my certification) provides a free week. Highland Yoga offers a month for $30 for new students at the time of this writing. Look for one of these franchises and try a beginner-friendly class offered at a studio near you.

Dedicating just a few minutes a day to yoga can lead to significant improvements in stress management and overall wellbeing.

Keep in mind you don't have to try all these suggestions at once. Pick one or two and see how your body responds in a week. You can take that a step further and write it down on your checklist to solidify it as part of your game plan. Keep what works and shelve the rest.

CHAPTER 3

Hack Your Hormone-Gut Connection

Simple Gut Health Protocol

It has been said that all disease starts in the gut. Well, did you know there is also a link between the health of your gut health and your hormone balance? Yep... More than 100 trillion diverse bacteria species exist in our gut, all of which we need for balanced gut health.

We call that bacterial population your microbiome. It develops at birth from your mother. This is part of your unique bio-individuality and helps regulate your estrogen levels through the "estrobolome." The estrobolome is a group of gut bacteria capable of metabolizing and regulating estrogen levels in the body.

However, an overgrowth of harmful bacteria in your gut can predispose you to a hormone imbalance. This means there's a disproportion between beneficial and detrimental bacterial species in your gastrointestinal tract.

This can be caused by our genes, diet choices—compromising proteins found in un-sprouted grains, sugar, genetically-modified foods (GMO), and dairy products—which can break down the gut lining or...

Even stress can completely change how the gut works. Do you ever get nervous or worried and feel butterflies in your stomach, or it induces a bowel movement? This is an example of the strong connection between anxiety, chronic stress, and GI issues.

Gut health affects the body's stress response, which in turn influences the production of stress hormones like cortisol. Chronic release of the hormone cortisol can also break down the gut barrier.

Large holes or cracks form when the gut barrier is compromised, allowing toxins, partly digested food, and gut bugs to penetrate the tissues beneath it. This is referred to as "Leaky Gut."

When toxins enter the bloodstream and reach other organs, they cause inflammation, impacting hormone regulation, including insulin signaling. It also presents in some people as an autoimmune disease like Hashimoto's thyroiditis. But for those without an autoimmune disease, we typically remain unaware that a leaky gut is the culprit.

Often the first signs are food sensitivities. For example, suddenly you can't eat wheat or dairy without gas or bloating. Maybe sugar cravings send you bouncing off the walls, and fiber makes you miserable. You may break out in hives, get a runny nose, or have debilitating headaches.

Often, simply removing the food culprit from your diet will have a huge impact on your health and provide immediate and dramatic results.

You have two options here. You can pay close attention to how your body responds after eating, or you can do a food sensitivity test. They are available online, and can even be done at home.

You can find some of my favorite at-home tests here:

www.amazon.com/shop/beastmom_fitnesshormonehacker

Now, let's focus on healing your gut!

The provided nutrition plan at the back of this book covers most dietary concerns, which can alleviate some symptoms. However, remember that there may be more you need to explore. This chapter will give you the knowledge to continue healing your body, reducing your symptoms, and aging gracefully long after you put this book down.

Remember, with any supplementation advice, please consult your healthcare provider first.

Add a Probiotic

Over time, the use of antibiotics, alcohol, poor diet, the impacts of stress, illness, and aging have led to shifts in this bacteria population. This decrease in gut flora makes the body more vulnerable. Any breakdown in the gut lining leads to a continuous source of infection and the long-term use of antibiotics causes resistant bacteria to overgrow.

Do you ever get sick, and a few weeks later you are sick again? Antibiotics could be a contributing factor.

Consider taking a probiotic when on a prescription antibiotic to help replenish the good bacteria.

Another reason I suggest a probiotic is because much of the meat we've consumed (until now) contains antibiotics that were fed to the animals, creating even more superbugs in our gut.

A quality probiotic can help reset your healthy gut microbiome. But buyer beware... not all probiotics are the same. Different strains offer different benefits. Common strains include Lactobacillus, Bifidobacterium, and Saccharomyces. It's often beneficial to choose a probiotic with a variety of strains.

Check the CFU Count. CFU stands for colony-forming units and indicates the number of live and active microorganisms in each dose. While there's no one-size-fits-all number, a general range to look for is between 1 billion to 10 billion CFUs for a daily supplement.

Pay attention to the storage instructions and expiration date. Some probiotics need to be refrigerated, while others are shelf-stable.

Begin with a lower dose and gradually increase it. This helps your body adjust to the probiotics without causing discomfort like bloating or gas.

For best results, take your probiotic regularly. But remember, noticing any changes or benefits might take a few weeks.

Everyone's body reacts differently. If you experience side effects or no improvement in your symptoms, consult a healthcare provider.

Especially if you have health issues or are on medication, it's important to talk to a healthcare provider before starting any new supplement, including probiotics.

Probiotics are generally considered safe, but they are not a one-size-fits-all solution. Tailoring your approach to your specific health needs and goals is critical.

What Meat Are You Eating?

The next step is to replace commercially raised meat in your diet with hormone and antibiotic free.

Remember earlier I mentioned that consumption of conventionally raised cattle means you are eating the hormones and antibiotics that the cattle were fed. That is why we are taking an extra step to cover all of our bases by choosing higher-quality proteins. Our bodies and the health of our hormones are worth the added expense.

Bone Broth

Drinking bone broth is one of the easiest ways to help heal your gut, along with dietary changes and stress relief. Its high content of amino acids like glutamine and collagen aids in the gut healing process. Glutamine supports gut lining integrity, helping to repair and maintain the mucosal lining of the gut. Collagen, which breaks down into gelatin during cooking, aids in soothing and protecting the gut lining. This approach can assist in diminishing inflammation and enhancing gut health.

Additionally, bone broth is easily digestible and can provide nutrients that support overall digestive health. You can purchase store-bought bone broth or make your own. Whenever I can, I make my own.

I've added a yummy bone broth recipe, so you always have something to sip on a couple times a week.

Organic Hormone-Free Bone Broth Recipe

Ingredients:

Bones: 2-3 pounds of mixed organic, hormone-free bones (beef, chicken, or turkey). Include a mix of marrow bones, joints, and meaty cuts for the best flavor and nutrient profile.

2 carrots, chopped

2 celery stalks, chopped

1 medium onion, chopped

4 garlic cloves, smashed

2 bay leaves

1 teaspoon whole black peppercorns

Fresh herbs like parsley or thyme (optional)

2 tbsp apple cider vinegar

Water, enough to cover bones by 2-3 inches (about 12-16 cups)

salt to taste (Himalayan pink or sea salt)

Instructions:

1. If beef bones are used, consider roasting them for 30 minutes at 400°F to enhance the flavor.

2. Rinse bones with cold water and pat them dry.

3. Place bones in a large stockpot or a slow cooker.

4. Add chopped vegetables, garlic, bay leaves, peppercorns, and any fresh herbs you use.

5. Pour in apple cider vinegar and add enough water to cover everything by a couple of inches.

6. Bring mixture to a gentle boil, then reduce heat to a simmer.

7. Allow to simmer for 12-24 hours. The longer it simmers, the richer and more nutritious it will be.

8. Skim off any foam that rises to the surface during the first few hours of simmering.

9. Strain broth through a fine-mesh sieve or cheesecloth to remove solids.

10. Let the broth cool, then transfer it to storage containers.

Refrigerate up to 5 days or freeze for longer storage.

Serving

Heat broth and season with salt to taste before serving.

Use as a base for soups, stews, or for cooking grains.

Nutritional Benefits:

Rich in minerals essential for bone health and overall wellness, like collagen and gelatin, which support skin health and joint mobility, and amino acids, which aid in gut health and immune system support.

Bone Broth Variations

Customizing your bone broth will not only enhance the flavor and also provide additional health benefits. Here is a short list of options:

Spices

Turmeric: Known for its anti-inflammatory properties. Remember to add a dash of pepper when using turmeric to activate the curcumin in it. Curcumin gives turmeric its antioxidant power.

Ginger: Fresh or powdered, ginger adds a warming flavor and aids digestion.

Cinnamon: A stick or a pinch of ground cinnamon can add a subtle sweetness and warmth.

Herbs

Rosemary: Adds a robust flavor and is known for its antioxidant properties.

Sage: Known for its potential to aid in cognitive function and memory, sage adds an earthy flavor.

Dandelion Greens: While not a traditional herb, these can be added for their potential liver-supportive properties.

Oils

Coconut Oil: A spoonful can add healthy fats and a subtle coconut flavor. Coconut oil regulates thyroid function.

Olive Oil: Drizzle in high-quality extra virgin olive oil after cooking for added heart-healthy fats.

Flaxseed Oil: Rich in omega-3 fatty acids, adding some flax seed oil can boost the nutritional profile.

Additional Options

Seaweed: For added minerals and a slight umami flavor, add kombu.

Lemongrass: For a refreshing and citrusy note.

Star Anise: Adds a licorice-like flavor and is good for digestion.

Experiment to find the combination that best suits your taste and health needs. Each ingredient contributes to the flavor profile and brings its own health benefits, making your bone broth a genuinely nourishing and therapeutic experience. Enjoy!!

Eat Fewer High-carb Foods

A diet high in processed carbs and low in nutrients can stress the gut lining, potentially leading to increased permeability ("leaky gut"). This can further disrupt hormonal balance by allowing substances into the bloodstream that can trigger immune and hormonal responses. Processed carbs, often high in sugar and low in fiber, can disrupt the balance of the gut microbiota. This imbalance can affect the metabolism of hormones like estrogen and cortisol.

Processed carbs also contribute to inflammation in the gut. Chronic inflammation can interfere with hormone regulation and signaling, including insulin, which is vital for blood sugar control.

You can instantly help your stomach by consuming less high-carbohydrate foods. Start by reducing sugar intake, white bread, juice, and French fries.

Add Fiber

Diets that are low in fiber and high in sugar are especially problematic. Consider adding some fiber to your daily meals.

Oats are a great option, at 16.5 grams of fiber per cup of raw oats.

Avocados provide 10 grams of fiber per cup and pack a punch with vitamin C, potassium, magnesium, E, and other B vitamins.

Lentils and kidney beans are also excellent sources of both fiber and protein.

Limit Highly Processed Foods

Avoid highly processed meats like sausage, hot dogs, and lunch meat. These are especially problematic for a healthy gut as they often contain gluten. And... have you seen how they're made? That's all I have to say about that!

White bread, margarine, and instant noodles are highly processed foods high in fat, salt, and sugar.

The Good News!

The good news is your body responds quickly to dietary changes, so following your nutrition plan and other weekly changes we make to help heal your body can lead to shifts in the gut that help you feel better right away.

After this program, as you continue on your path of optimal health and longevity, remember to:

- Drink bone broth
- Decrease sugar intake
- Increase fiber

- Improve the quality of meat and fat you consume

Simple changes can have a massive impact and improve your overall quality of life.

Autoimmune Conditions

Sometimes even after dietary and lifestyle changes, you may still experience symptoms. This is especially common if you have an autoimmune condition. In most cases you may not know an autoimmune condition is the problem. If this is the case for you, strongly consider speaking with your doctor, and DO NOT TAKE your results are "normal" as an answer. Often, these "normal" results are taken from measurements of a bunch of sick people. We don't want "normal," we want *optimal*. Ask to run a full thyroid panel (T3, T4, reverse T3, free T3 and free T4, tsh, and tpo the antibodies). This should give you and your doctor a clearer picture of what is going on in your body. Depending on your medical insurance, getting all of these tests run may be challenging. But this is one of those times when standing firm and advocating for your health matters. You can always visit a private lab and have your doctor review those results if necessary.

Questions You Can Ask Yourself

If you think there may be a gut issue and are not ready to test, here are a few questions to consider and a simple place to start.

- What physical digestive symptoms do I feel?

- Do I have any symptoms that aren't related to digestion, such as hives, headaches, or a runny nose?

- What foods have I eaten that I might have an allergy or sensitivity to?

I recommend keeping a weekly food journal to help pinpoint which foods might be responsible for any symptoms. From there, try eliminating suspicious foods for a week to see if symptoms improve.

Be sure to remove only one food at a time to pinpoint exactly where the sensitivity resides.

Observe How You Feel

What happens if you take the offending food out for a week?

Are there any shifts in your physical or emotional health?

If you think your gut issues might be stress-related, refer to the stress chapter for a list of stress-busting techniques to help you keep your gut in check.

Meet Mercedes, a dedicated nurse who faced the dual challenges of Graves' disease (an autoimmune condition) and perimenopause. Despite these hurdles, she achieved a remarkable transformation, shedding over 33 pounds, revitalizing her energy levels, and significantly reducing her medication dosage — not just once, but twice. This journey wasn't just about weight loss; it was a path to regaining her self-esteem and confidence, all thanks to our hormone-hacking program.

"Before joining the program, I was battling weight gain due to my Graves' medication. I felt perpetually exhausted, and my self-confidence had plummeted. Despite my efforts, including three-weekly HIIT classes, the scale refused to budge," recounts Mercedes.

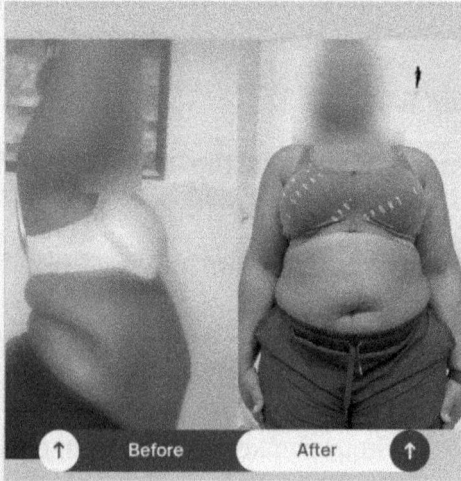

Her turning point came when she discovered our program. We crafted a hormone-balancing nutrition plan and lifestyle adjustments uniquely tailored to her needs. We focused on restoring her gut by removing known offenders like dairy, gluten and soy and adding in quality probiotics to replenish the good gut bacteria. The outcome was nothing short of remarkable.

Mercedes not only lost over 33 pounds but also experienced a resurgence in her energy and a significant boost in her confidence. Her medication dosage was successfully reduced twice, bringing it to the lowest level she's ever been on. "I feel sexy again," she exclaims with a radiant smile.

We are overjoyed with her success and honored to have played a role in her journey. Mercedes' story is a testament to the transformative power of personalized care and support.

She remains one of our most cherished nurse clients, who not only overcame weight gain and fatigue during perimenopause but also conquered self-sabotage. Through our specialized hormone-balancing nutrition plan, personalized lifestyle changes, and dedicated coaching, Mercedes rediscovered her zest for life.

Now that you have an understanding of how gut health impacts your hormones and your overall health, use this Simple Gut Health Protocol as a guide to address minor gut and digestive issues.

Start by introducing one or two of the steps outlined in the protocol this week, then add more as you get comfortable with the current practices. Use the checklist provided to ensure you have a simple game plan to follow moving forward.

It could be as simple as adding probiotics this week and removing some processed carbs.

In many cases, a little goes a long way in improving gut function!

When deciding what foods to eat, consider how you want to feel.

My mission is to empower you to defy the social norms on aging so you achieve your wellness, fitness and body goals... no matter what. I have helped countless women snatch those waists, get rid of hot flashes, brain fog, and night sweats. It's your turn!

Need an accountability buddy so you don't feel so alone? Join our Free Facebook community of like-minded women on the same journey.

www.facebook.com/groups/hormonehackingandnaturalfatloss

Chapter 4

Hack Your Fitness

During my 30s, I began experiencing the early signs of perimenopause. My weight was on an upward trend, sleep became elusive, and I heavily indulged in alcohol. Desperate for a solution, I experimented with various diets and quick fixes like the cabbage soup diet, B12 injections, and phentermine... Yes phentermine. I can't believe that it's legal. These efforts were primarily futile, offering only temporary relief before I regained the lost weight, often with additional pounds.

Self-sabotage was also a constant battle, but I reached a point where enough was enough. My education in nutrition opened my eyes to the power of eating for hormonal balance. I eliminated alcohol, focused on the quality of the meats and produce I consumed, and cut down on processed foods. I incorporated a high-quality multivitamin, omega-3s, and a reliable probiotic into my routine, and made sure to get enough rest. I also embraced weightlifting and cardio, and was amazed at the positive changes in how I felt. This inspired me to help other women like myself and become an amateur fitness competitor.

Gone were the weekends of alcohol and takeout. I no longer missed that dreadful feeling after a night of heavy drinking and consuming loads of processed foods. It's true what they say: once you experience true wellness, you realize how accustomed you had become to feeling unwell, and that's not what living should be.

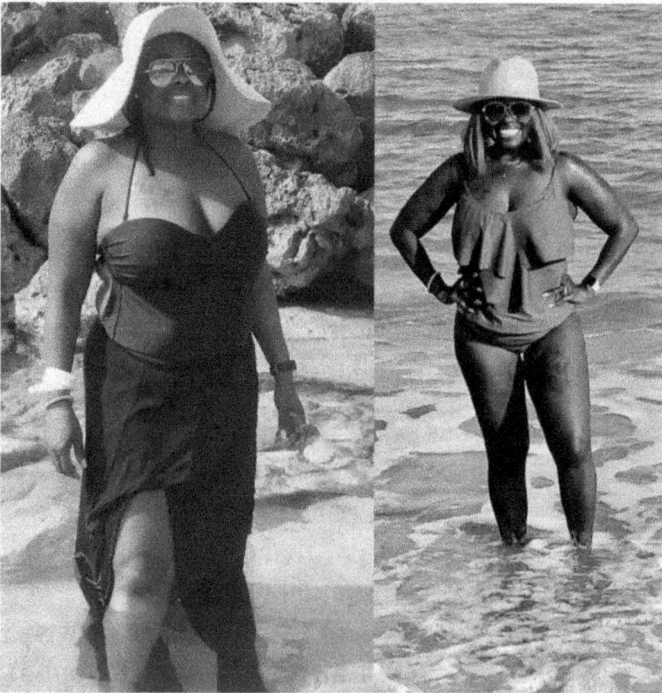

Our diet shouldn't leave us feeling bloated, lethargic, overheated, or in pain. It should make us feel light, satisfied, and full of energy. If your experience is anything but this, it's time to reevaluate what you're putting into your body. I lost over 45 pounds, regained my confidence, and no longer hid my body from my husband.

Your Fitness Goals

If you're reading this, chances are you're either beginning, eager to start, or resuming your fitness journey!

You might be aiming to:

- Gain confidence in social outings with friends

- Boost your energy for meaningful family time

- Slip comfortably into your "goal" jeans

- Overcome breathlessness or fatigue when climbing stairs

Or it could be a blend of these goals. Embarking on this journey can seem daunting at first. You may question whether your approach is correct or if it will be effective. Moreover, you might find your mind attempting to dissuade you from starting. Rest assured, you're in the right place.

This chapter will lay out the basics you need to know.

I want to help you take those first few steps in a fun way, empowering, and (best of all!) *effective!*

This is why I advise getting an OK from your doctor or healthcare provider before you start *any* new workout or nutrition program.

Ready to jump in? Great... let's GET STARTED!

Three Pillars of Fitness

There are three essential components of everyday fitness. It's important to include all of them in your exercise regimen for optimal results.

1 STRENGTH

This is about more than building big muscles (which is more complicated than most people think!).

On a practical level, it's about possessing the strength to effortlessly perform everyday activities in life. This is what keeps us out of nursing homes: fitness for function.

It also can include being able to pick up heavy things just for fun, if you want... like your kids or grandkids... lol. Strength training also helps increase the body's production of testosterone... (yes, ladies, we make testosterone too) which increases fat burning and increases libido.

Minimum Recommendations:

At least two days a week, do a muscle-strengthening workout that targets all of your major muscle groups (chest, back, shoulders, legs, arms). Or you can split it up doing upper and lower body on separate days.

This can include bodyweight exercises, machine weights, resistance bands, free weights, kettlebells, suspension trainers, or other equipment.

2 ENDURANCE & STAMINA

This is commonly known as cardio and it's the kind of exercise most associated with the mood-boosting endorphin "rush."

For health benefits, you should get at least 150 minutes (2.5 hours) of moderate intensity or 75 minutes of vigorous exercise (or a combo of the two) over the course of a week. It's better if you spread this out.

That may sound like a lot, but it's only 30 minutes a day for 5 days a week.

That being said, you get even *more* health benefits if you work out more. (I recommend building up the amount over time, though.) For me, four 45-minute cardio sessions a week is plenty, and it's usually a mix of HIIT cardio and strength training.

And you guessed it! Sample cardio workouts are included here in this chapter.

Smart tip: It's a good idea to get into basic cardio shape before you add any vigorous activity (i.e., you should be able to jog before you start sprinting!).

3 FLEXIBILITY & MOBILITY

You should do flexibility and mobility exercises (like stretching or yoga) for all major muscle groups (shoulders, chest, back, hips, legs) at least 2 to 3 times a week. This doesn't have to take long, either, as 10-minute stretching sessions are fine.

Just a few benefits:

- Having supple, flexible muscles can reduce your risk of injury

- Having "looser" muscles can equal fewer aches and pains

- Better posture and balance

- Improved performance

You'll find a sample stretching routine at the end of this chapter that you can do on its own or after other workouts.

Super Savvy Tip

Download your FREE copy of
my beautiful, full-color
Beastmom Beginner's Guide to Fitness:

Hackyourhormonesforweightloss.com/bonuses

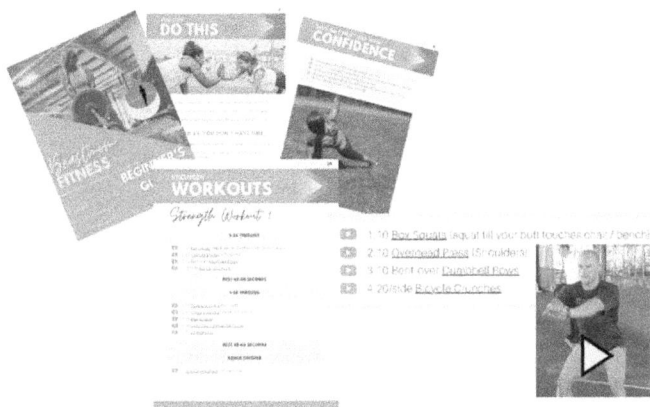

14-Day Beginner Exercise Guide

This routine is just a guideline. Listen to your body. If your muscles are extremely sore, take an extra rest day or go for a walk. Add the stretching routine after 2 to 3 of your workouts each week.

NOTE: Always consult your physician or other healthcare provider before starting any exercise program.

Week 1

DAY 1	DAY 2	DAY 3	DAY 4	DAY 5	DAY 6	DAY 7
Walk or steady-state cardio	Strength workout 1	Walk & stretches	Do anywhere cardio HIIT	Rest	Strength workout 2	Interval walk or cardio

Week 2

DAY 8	DAY 9	DAY 10	DAY 11	DAY 12	DAY 13	DAY 14
Rest	Strength workout 1	Walk & stretches	Do anywhere cardio HIIT	Rest	Strength workout 2	Interval walk or cardio

28-Day Beginner Workout

Week 1

DAY 1	DAY 2	DAY 3	DAY 4	DAY 5	DAY 6	DAY 7
Walk or steady-state cardio	Quick total body	Walk/run & stretches	Leg HIIT	Rest	Total Body Metabolic challenge	Interval walk or cardio

Week 2

DAY 8	DAY 9	DAY 10	DAY 11	DAY 12	DAY 13	DAY 14
Rest	Amrap	Walk/run & stretches	Arm and abs HIIT	Rest	Bodyweight conditioning	Interval walk or cardio

Week 3

DAY 1	DAY 2	DAY 3	DAY 4	DAY 5	DAY 6	DAY 7
Walk or steady-state cardio	Quick total body	Walk/run & stretches	Leg HIIT	Rest	Total Body Metabolic challenge	Interval walk or cardio

Week 4

DAY 8	DAY 9	DAY 10	DAY 11	DAY 12	DAY 13	DAY 14
Rest	Amrap	Walk/run & stretches	Arm and abs HIIT	Rest	Bodyweight conditioning	Interval walk or cardio

Strength Workouts

All you need for these workouts are some dumbbells – light enough to do each exercise with great form but heavy enough to feel a little challenging by the last repetition! And if you can do more than 12 reps without feeling a burn, increase your weights by about 10 percent until you get there.

If you don't have a bench for some exercises, find a sturdy table, aerobics step, counter, or other platform.

Warm up with light cardio before beginning these workouts.

Do grouped exercises back-to-back, take a 45 to 60-second break, and repeat 2-3 times. Then, move on to the next group of exercises.

Strength Workout 1

1-3X THROUGH

- ❖ 10 Box Squats
  (Squat till your butt touches chair / bench)

- ❖ 10 Overhead Press *(Shoulders)*

- ❖ 10 Bent-over Dumbbell Rows

- ❖ 20/side Bicycle Crunches

REST 45-60 SECONDS

1-3X THROUGH

- ❖ 10 Reverse Lunges each side

- ❖ 10 Incline Pushups (hands on bench)

- ❖ 10 Biceps Curls

- ❖ 10 Overhead Triceps Extensions

- ❖ 15 Glute Bridge

REST 45-60 SECONDS

BONUS FINISHER

- ❖ Straight-Arm Plank, 30 seconds

Strength Workout 2

1-3X THROUGH

- ❖ 12 Bodyweight Squats

- ❖ 12 Triceps Dips

- ❖ 12 Dumbbell Hammer Curl

- ❖ 20-second Side Plank (from knee) per side

REST 45-60 SECONDS

1-3X THROUGH

- ❖ 12 Braced Single-Leg Romanian deadlift
  (hand on bench for support)

- ❖ 12 Dumbbell Chest Press

- ❖ 12 Reverse Flies

- ❖ 12 Bird Dogs

REST 45-60 SECONDS

BONUS FINISHER

- ❖ Alphabet Plank! *(In a forearm plank position, spell the alphabet with your belly button, resting as often as needed, until you complete the alphabet.)*

Cardio Workouts

WALKING

Walking for fitness means picking up the pace! Be purposeful and have intention with your stride and posture.

If you are not used to walking, ramp up your speed and duration over the course of a couple weeks.

Goal: Walk at a pace of 3 to 4 miles an hour and aim to match or exceed that distance in the same amount of time or less for each walk once you get acclimated.

STEADY-STATE CARDIO

Warm up for 3-5 minutes, then keep a steady pace for 20 to 45 minutes.

You should be working hard enough to still easily carry on a conversation but not be able to sing without getting out of breath.

These workouts are good energy and mood boosters. You're guaranteed to work up a sweat!

TIP: Create a great music playlist to keep you motivated.

INTERVAL CARDIO
(great for fat-burning and testosterone production)

Warm up for 5-7 minutes, then pick up the pace for anywhere from 30 seconds to 2 minutes. Then take an active "recovery" break by slowing down for 30 seconds to 2 minutes, and repeat.

Alternate periods of hard/easy work for 20-30 minutes, then cool down for 5-7 minutes so your heart rate returns to normal.

TIP: Listen to your body during these workouts. If you are new to exercising, or are coming back after a layoff, establish a good baseline of fitness before attempting high-effort intervals.

DO-ANYWHERE METABOLIC CONDITIONING / HIIT

This is no-equipment workout will strengthen your body while keeping your heart rate up and burning more fat than steady-state cardio!

Warm up with a brisk walk or other cardio exercise for 5-7 minutes. Then perform this circuit, taking breaks between exercises and 30 to 60 seconds rest between circuit rounds.

- ❖ 15 Jumping Jacks
  (low impact – touch right foot to side then left foot)
  (high impact – jumping)
  Low impact is best for women with high cortisol

- ❖ 5 Pushups

- ❖ 10 Reverse Lunges each side

- ❖ 10 Bicycle Crunches each side

- ❖ 10 Squats

- ❖ 10 Mountain Climbers
  (keep core engaged – Option: do with hands elevated)

REST 45-60 SECONDS

REPEAT for total of 15-20 MINUTES

COOL DOWN: 5-10 MINUTES of WALKING

Flexibility Workout

STRETCHING WORKOUT

To get the most out of your stretches, perform them after walking or other exercise that warms up your muscles.

This will help you stretch through a wider range of motion.

> HOLD EACH STRETCH FOR 30-60 SECONDS

- ❖ Chest stretch

- ❖ Quadriceps stretch

- ❖ Hamstring stretch

- ❖ Cat-Cow stretch

- ❖ Hip/Glute stretch

- ❖ Figure 4 stretch

- ❖ Hip flexor stretch

BONUS TIPS FOR BEST RESULTS

❖ Eat a small snack about an hour before your strength workouts.

❖ Stay hydrated! Make sure you drink water during or after your workout.

During the first few workouts is NOT the time to pick up heavy weights or go all-out. Let your body adjust to exercise first to avoid injury and excessive soreness. Then, later on, you can ramp up the intensity.

Follow this routine and you'll feel stronger, fitter, and more energized – and best of all, you will be on your way to creating a HEALTHY LIFESTYLE that can last a lifetime!

Grab your checklist and decide how many workouts you will commit to this week and what they will be. It can be as simple as one cardio, one strength, and one stretching. You can build from there.

Chapter 5

Weight-loss Triggers That Work While You Sleep

I already know what you're thinking. *But Phyllis, ever since menopause, I can't sleep anymore!*

I hear you. That oh-so-elusive 8 hours of sleep.... Where the heck is it? That is the question many women in menopause are asking.

But sleep troubles aren't exclusive to women in menopause. In my thirties, I started having sleep troubles. That was the first sign that I was beginning perimenopause. My first thought was, *Oh my God... my youth is over!* Then I went on a quest to find out how to fix it.

Changes in hormone levels can lead to various physical and emotional symptoms. One of the most common is sleep disturbances or insomnia. Hot flashes and night sweats are also common symptoms that interfere with sleep.

In addition to hormonal changes, it is reported that women over 40 tend to be more highly stressed. And guess what... increased stress and anxiety can also affect sleep quality. Here's the kicker...when we are highly stressed, our bodies will take progesterone (our keep-calm hormone) to make more cortisol. This can be a vicious cycle.

When the stuff of daily life never turns off or lets you hit the pause button, it makes it harder to get proper rest.

Your body can't distinguish when it is under mental or physical stress either, and it instantly prioritizes the production of cortisol—our stress hormone. This makes it harder to sleep at night, lowering the production of melatonin—our sleep hormone.

The result is you lie awake at night, unable to sleep because the cortisol puts your body on high alert... it's telling your body to stay awake so it can be on the lookout for threats.

No big surprise here, but not getting enough sleep can halt and even reverse your weight-loss efforts.

Of course there seems to be no end of stressful things in our lives at this age. We're worried about our weight, we're worried about our kids, we're worried about our spouses, and we're even worried about our aging parents. Continuous stress disrupts sleep, removing all the tools you have to solve those worries—your energy, your motivation, and your mind.

Poor sleep also weakens the immune system. It drives up your appetite, increases blood pressure, and worsens depression.

A single night of inadequate sleep can reduce insulin sensitivity by 33 percent, throwing off our hunger hormones, ghrelin and leptin. This is why when we're sleep-deprived we make poor food choices. When your insulin is not regulated, it can lead to symptoms like dizziness, hunger, sweating, a faster heart rate, trouble concentrating, and blurred vision. Sleep is critical to maintaining your insulin levels and regulating all of the other hormones affected by insulin.

Insulin resistance is the result of chronic reduced insulin sensitivity. This is when your muscles, fat, and liver cells react poorly to insulin and struggle to absorb glucose from your blood effectively. As a result, your pancreas has to work harder to make more insulin to help glucose enter your cells.

Insulin resistance is part of the problem when we struggle to eliminate that belly fat. And if you have a thyroid disorder, it's a double whammy.

This perfectly explains why poor sleep is associated with weight gain.

Have you ever noticed that it's harder to resist cookies and other sweets at the office after a night of poor sleep?

Continuous poor sleep can cause declines in many areas if not remedied. How can you get to the root causes behind what's keeping you awake so you can benefit from all the good stuff that sleep offers? Well, let's talk about that...

Your body functions on signals and rhythms. It manages sleep on a circadian rhythm—physical, mental, and behavioral signals that follow a 24-hour cycle. Therefore, creating or resetting your daily patterns will help regulate sleep and wakefulness.

Light is what triggers this system to function properly. When light decreases, as it does at night, a hormone called melatonin is released, which results in sleepiness. When light increases, as it does in the morning, melatonin decreases, shifting you into a state of wakefulness.

It sounds simple, but our modern world has made this process increasingly difficult. Thanks to electricity, televisions, and smartphones, we stay connected and in brightly lit environments more hours than ever.

Lack of sleep is perceived by your body as stress. That alone triggers a stress response, releasing cortisol. When your body prioritizes making cortisol, it de-prioritizes producing melatonin—our sleep hormone—and our thyroid hormone, which you need to regulate your metabolism (along with many other processes in the body) which is your fat-burning system.

So take a second and wrap your head around what you just learned. When you aren't sleeping, your hormones, or lack thereof, make you eat. On top of that, the lack of sleep increases cortisol production, reducing your body's production of thyroid hormone, which regulates your metabolism. That's how not sleeping contributes to weight gain and hormone imbalances.

The Solutions

Enough doom and gloom. Let's talk solutions!

With these action steps in place, you'll be able to supercharge your sleep. That way you can stop struggling against cravings, a slowed metabolism, irregular appetite, insulin resistance, and even brain fog.

Bedtime

So you can benefit from all the effort you're putting into hormone balance and losing weight, you need to prioritize quality sleep.

A consistent sleep routine is far more critical when experiencing hormonal change. Going to bed at the same time each night and waking up at the same time each morning makes a huge difference. Even if you aren't falling asleep, you're basically sleep-training your body... just like we do with a baby.

Your Sleep Environment

Developing a regular sleep pattern creates a space conducive to good sleep. Beyond keeping a regular bedtime, there are simple changes you can make to your bedroom that increase the likelihood of you getting the quality sleep you deserve.

Make your sleeping environment completely dark. Opt for light-blocking curtains.

Remove electronics, which emit light and radio frequencies that can disturb sleep.

Get a comfortable pillow-top mattress cover and quality high thread-count sheets. You could also indulge in an oversized soft comforter and nice-smelling candles.

I have a lavender-infused mattress topper and soft night lights in my bedroom. I also turn on classical music that is on a timer to help me drift off to sleep.

Find out what works for you that is soothing and rewarding. Every step you take to make your bedroom a welcoming and relaxing space contributes to an aura of self-care and pampering.

Don't think of this as selfish! When you are sleep-deprived, you are less able to take care of your loved ones. If you feel like you're carrying the weight of the world, trick yourself into making your sleep a priority because it will help you better serve others.

Things to Avoid Before Bedtime

Be sure you are working out no less than two hours before bed... unless it's gentle yoga. Intense exercise too close to bedtime will increase cortisol levels disturbing your sleep.

Also avoid eating for several hours before bedtime. When you eat, it activates the digestive system, which disturbs sleep. Try to finish eating at least 2 to 3 hours before bed.

Avoid caffeine too late in the day. For me, that means no coffee after 3:00 PM, and no more than two cups daily. Coffee reduces melatonin production... our sleep hormone. As a first step, try replacing some of that coffee with half-decaf as you work on cutting back.

Believe it or not, alcohol also disturbs sleep. While it may make you fall asleep faster, it interferes with REM sleep, which is when most people dream. This stage of sleep is crucial for getting adequate rest and supporting your adrenal glands—which during the hormonal change years is essential for hormone balance, metabolizing fat, and daytime wakefulness. Alcohol also increases instances of sleep apnea, which is when a person stops breathing during sleep.

Finally, use the features on your phone to automatically switch to nighttime settings. It's no secret that the blue light emitted from cell phones, tablets, computers, and TV suppresses melatonin. Even reading on your device can make it take longer for you to fall asleep.

The night shift feature on your devices applies a filter that limits the blue light emitted. Additionally, you can dim the screen to avoid glare.

Activate the Bedtime (iOS) or Wind Down (Android) feature that allows you to set a bedtime after which all notifications are silenced for the night.

For best practice, put aside your cell phone and all digital devices 45 minutes before bed.

Create a Nightly Ritual

A soothing bedtime routine sets the stage for a good night's sleep. As mentioned before, your body runs on signals. Your body also needs a signal at bedtime, but it doesn't have to be complicated.

It can be as simple as reading a good book right before sleep. For me it's my herbal tea, lavender on my hands and pillow, and a mindless activity to unwind. Create a wind-down routine that stops screen time and focuses on mental and physical relaxation.

Install light dimmers in your home on a timer, and set them to start dimming an hour or two before bed. That signals to your body that it is time to wind down.

Use this time to pamper yourself... Put on some tea and soft music, and run a hot Epsom salt bath. Whatever makes it quiet time in your home.

This also sets an amazing example for your kids to put away electronics and be present with one another as you set the stage for a restful night of sleep. I am not saying this will be easy, but your body needs the wind down.

Try this alternate nostril breathing technique if you deal with a high-stress life. WebMD recommends this easy method:

> Place your thumb over your right nostril. With this nostril blocked, close your eyes and exhale thoroughly and slowly through your left nostril.

> Once you've exhaled completely, release your right nostril, and put your ring finger on the left nostril. Breathe in deeply and slowly from the right side.

While you obviously shouldn't practice this while driving, operating machinery, or anything else that requires concentration, this kind of breathing helps regulate the nervous system, lowers blood pressure, and improves breathing. It can also help lower fear and anxiety, and who doesn't need that?

Another option is a natural sleep aid. At the time of this writing, I alternate between natural drops from Sprouts called iSleep, which has several herbs including valerian root and melatonin. On other nights I take something called Rest zzz's, also from Sprouts, which has passionflower, chamomile, valerian, melatonin and GABA. I also recommend looking into time-released melatonin. As with all supplements... discuss it with your healthcare provider first and read the labels. Some low-cost supplements include fillers like gluten or soy, which can work against our hormone-balancing efforts.[1]

Try taking a hot bath with lavender Epsom salts, and lavender or other calming essential oils, with soft music playing and candles. A hot aromatherapy shower can also do the trick.

Consider adding a relaxing habit like meditation, journaling, or gentle stretching to your bedtime ritual. You might enjoy "Yoga with Adriene" on YouTube. In addition to her 10 and 20-minute yoga for bedtime offerings, she has wind-down routines and stretching specific to body parts that might be causing you pain.

---

[1] Be sure to read the labels of any supplements you buy. You want to be sure they haven't added unnecessary additives, especially soy.

Bedtime Beverage

Finally, I'd like to share a recipe that I love.

When it comes to bedtime, herbal tea is a great option. I love passionflower and chamomile tea because they give me a bit of sweetness and help relax me before bed. Passionflower is known for its sleep and anti-anxiety qualities.

One of my favorite tea additions is flavored magnesium. However, I have found that my body gets used to it over time and it no longer helps, so cycling on and off seems to resolve that problem.

I have also added lemon balm, ashwagandha[2], and magnesium glycinate to my bedtime tea.

But sometimes you just want something a little richer and more comforting! This recipe is a perfect match. It's warm, relaxing, and has a flavor reminiscent of a spice cookie! (Seriously.) Plus, it's packed with ingredients aimed at helping you combat stress and fall asleep quicker.

While the spice mix may seem daunting, don't let that deter you. These spices are easily found in grocery stores and offer numerous health benefits.

---

[2] Consult a doctor before using ashwagandha, as it can react with some prescription medications.

Cinnamon aids in stabilizing your blood sugar, turmeric effectively reduces inflammation, and nutmeg is rich in sleep-promoting phytonutrients.

If you enjoy this recipe as much as I do, it'll become a staple of your nightly routine. Consider preparing the spice mix in larger quantities for convenience whenever you wish to use it. A serving is about 2 teaspoons of the bulk-prepared blend, but feel free to adjust this to suit your taste.

Golden Moon Milk

- 1 cup (240 ml) unsweetened cashew, almond or hemp milk
- ½ tsp ground cinnamon
- ½ tsp ground turmeric
- ¼ tsp ground ginger
- ¼ tsp ground cardamom
- Pinch of ground nutmeg
- Pinch of ground clove
- Freshly ground black pepper
- ¼ tsp ground ashwagandha (optional)[3]
- 1 tsp melted coconut oil
- 1 tsp raw honey (optional)

---

[3] The recipe is just fine without ashwagandha, so no worries if you can't find this ingredient or don't want to use it because of concerns about pairing it with other prescription medications!

Bring the nut milk to a simmer in a small saucepan over medium-low heat. While that's heating, in a small bowl whisk together all the spices and ashwagandha (if you're using it).

Next, whisk the spices into the milk, making sure to dissolve any clumps. Add the coconut oil, lower the heat, and cook for 7-10 minutes.

Remove the saucepan from the heat and let it cool slightly before adding the honey.

Pour into a mug and enjoy!

Note: I don't use honey because this recipe is pretty sweet as is, but feel free to adjust this to your taste. Organic maple syrup would make a nice variation, too.

One of my former clients, Dee, has a pretty demanding work schedule.

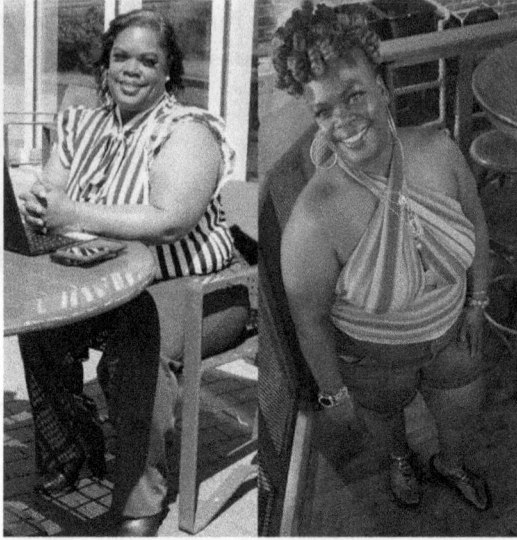

Along with dialing in her nutrition so her blood sugar stayed balanced, we worked on weekly sleep goals. Dee drank my herbal sleep tea which helped her get better sleep and her energy back. She's now down over 30 pounds. The improved sleep, energy, and weight loss are massive accomplishments for a hypothyroid client!

Incorporate 1 or 2 of the great techniques from this chapter to hack your hormones for weight loss while you sleep by adding it to your checklist!

Chapter 6

Functional Medicine Agrees

It's tempting to give up when you're doing everything "right," and still, the weight doesn't come off. The culprit could be your hormones. I want you to have more information to finally get your desired results.

I interviewed Dr. Sharleen Lawrence to confirm what I've been sharing with you. Dr. Sharleen is a licensed acupuncturist, a certified Functional Medicine Practitioner, and a Certified Hypnotherapist who practices in Southern California.

You'll see the questions I asked her in bold below, followed by Dr. Sharleen's answers.

Do hormones actually affect weight loss?

Absolutely! I've been helping women hack their hormones for about nine years. From the thyroid hormones to the sex hormones, these are the chemical messengers of the body's adrenal system. It's all intertwined. Once something goes astray, it typically sends a ton of other things out of balance.

I specialize in Hashimoto's disease, which is a thyroid hormone problem. Women get triggered during the three P's—puberty, pregnancy, and perimenopause—and it brings substantial hormone changes. So if we're looking at weight loss without factoring in the hormones, you're missing a huge part of the pie.

Do you think that trouble losing weight could be a symptom of a hormone imbalance?

Yes, I get people coming in all the time. They say, "I've tried everything... I've done fasting. I've worked out two hours a day, six days a week. But I either stay the same or put on more weight." That's because the hormones shift after age 35. And it can happen even earlier than that. If your nutrition is dialed in, you're exercising and getting in your steps three to five times a week, but you're not losing weight, the first place you need to look is hormones.

For women who take thyroid medication, if you push yourself harder in the gym, you're making your thyroid condition worse. If you restrict calories, you're making your thyroid condition worse. The things we were taught when we were younger—eat less and move more—are not good advice anymore.

So many people today have adrenal fatigue, in which case moving more may not be sound advice for that person. Fasting is not useful in Hashimoto's or a hypothyroid condition. It's actually counterproductive. Fasting is really complicated, depending on what stage of life you are at and how your hormones fluctuate.

At the same time, your husband can drop weight just by giving up cookies. Maybe you haven't eaten in four days, but you're still packing on the weight. It's so frustrating! These women ask, "What am I doing wrong?" The hormones are just working differently in women's bodies. It's also possible to have a thyroid condition and not even know it. With the hormonal shift, whether it be perimenopause or menopause, that often triggers a thyroid condition.

What foods can we eat to help us lose weight and get our hormones in balance?

Let's start with what I think you shouldn't eat. Most people would do well by avoiding the Big Six: gluten, dairy, soy, caffeine, alcohol, and sugar.

Of course every time I share this list, someone says, "Oh my god, there's no way I could give up dairy... or bread... or whatever it is." I promise you, if I can do it, you can do it. But if you're someone who thinks those six are essential to life, I recommend you start by shopping the perimeter of the grocery store—produce, meat, eggs. Just skip over the dairy and see what happens. You might notice your skin gets better, you have less bloating and gas, less brain fog.

The proteins, especially if you're vegan or vegetarian, are a little more challenging, for sure. Still, you can find amazing recipes with fruits, veggies, and higher-quality meats if it's in your budget. Try to get organic grass-fed meats and pasture-raised chicken and eggs. You want those deep golden yolks inside that look orange.

Avoiding those center aisles gets you away from so many products that contain soy. Even the gluten-free stuff has soy in it. Those center-aisle products might be chock full of omega-6 fatty acids, which we need, but we need them in smaller quantities and certain ratios with the omega-3s. Plus all of those vegetable oils and corn oils create tons of inflammation in the body. Adding inflammation on top of a hormone imbalance on top of adrenal fatigue... you're just a mess. Inflammation also exacerbates problems for those with an autoimmune condition.

When patients start reading the labels, they're surprised to see how many of the foods they eat contain gluten and soy. They say, "Oh my god, everything?"

I have a Hashimoto patient who has reluctantly given up gluten and dairy. Her daughter is doing it with her... and the daughter is getting amazing results! But she's not, because she refuses to give up processed foods, which are full of soy. She says, "I just won't do it." I reply, "Well, you told me you want to feel better. You spend a lot of money coming to see me, but you won't do this simple thing?" It's all about balance. We have to find what's right for us. And what I find is that sometimes we forget what it feels like to feel good. Until we feel good, we can't compare it to how crappy we felt before we got rid of these foods.

Sometimes the pain just isn't deep enough for them to change!

How do I know which hormones are out of balance?

This can be tricky. As a functional medicine practitioner, I love to test, not guess. But at the same time, certain symptoms do point to specific hormones, so if you're not in a position to get the testing, you can at least start biohacking yourself.

Fatigue is the top symptom if you think you have a thyroid issue. This is a level of fatigue where you always have to nap in the afternoon now, but even just a couple of years ago, you never had to do that. Hair falling out is a big sign, as is gaining weight all over the body. This is a big red flag for thyroid issues, because every single cell in the body uses thyroid hormone. So literally anywhere in the body can go out of whack when you have a thyroid problem.

For female patients, especially if they still have a cycle, breast tenderness—either around ovulation time or when their cycle is coming—can point to estrogen dominance. You might want to look at bringing estrogen down by taking something like a DIM (Di-Indolyl Methane) supplement.

Make sure to get your supplements from a provider and not Costco or CVS, because those have gluten fillers and are junk. Third-party certification is better... the bargain brands are bargain for a reason! But they really aren't a bargain... because you've invested all of this money but they're not doing what you intend to do.

If you are that person your family can't stand to be around for those couple of days leading up to your cycle, your progesterone could be off.

If you used to love sex but now, a couple years down the road or after having kids, you're like, "Don't ever look at me or touch me again," testosterone might be to blame.

These are just some classic signs and symptoms that might lead to certain hormones, but testing is the best way to find out where you are. You want to look at things like your DHEA and FSH, which will determine whether or not you're post-menopausal. Look at all three types of estrogen, because often the doctors just run estradiol tests. There's also estriol and estrone. Also look at progesterone, prolactin, testosterone, and possibly even cortisol.

Not all doctors run a full panel because of insurance limitations. That's where functional medicine practitioners come into play... when you genuinely want to see the whole picture. With thyroid, I actually run 10 different markers.

As a woman, you want to see where your testosterone is, because DHEA is the precursor to all the sex hormones. Suppose DHEA isn't converting properly into testosterone. In that case, that means you're going to have muscle wasting—it's going to be hard to build muscle, your energy is gonna be low, bones get weaker, and you'll feel like you don't want to have sex ever again. Testosterone keeps us vibrant.

Any final recommendations?

Know your body and pay attention to what it's telling you. If you've been gaslighted by doctors, keep advocating for yourself because there are solutions out there. You don't have to be fat, tired, and called lazy... because you're not. You have great people in your corner like Phyllis and myself. Just keep advocating for yourself and you will find the answers.

If your test results are normal, but you know something is off, don't just leave the office. We aren't shooting for normal. We're shooting for optimal! Keep asking for what you need, or reach out to someone who will listen.

Great advice from Dr. Sharleen! It's affirming to know that you're not the only one this happens to, and are not imagining things. Finding someone who listens to you is critical. Having great support as you hack your hormones, your stress, your nutrition, and your fitness is vital!

If nutrition and lifestyle change doesn't seem to be enough... reach out to me for customized help and coaching at:

Phyllis@hackyourhormonesforweightloss.com

CHAPTER 7

Bringing It All Together....

You're starting the new year in a different headspace with a new mission and energy to go after it. So let's put it together in a daily goal sheet/checklist for you to follow.

Step 1: We are going to set a goal. But not just any goal—a S.M.A.R.T goal. I know you've seen that acronym before, but the provided checklist will help you put it into practice.

We want your goals to be Specific, like:

- Lose 8-10 pounds this month

- Improve my energy

- Better quality of life

We want your goals to be Measurable and Attainable. Refrain from setting goals so large that you set yourself up for failure. For example, 8-10 pounds could be an achievable goal for one month.

We want to give our goals a timeline. Set your one-month goal and then use those numbers to create an overall goal and the number of months it would realistically take. For example: "I want to lose 24-30 pounds in the next four months."

Then you want to write down your "BIG WHY." This has to be bigger than "I want to lose weight to look good naked." That's a good reason, but you need something to motivate you to make better choices on those tough days.

For example, it could be:

"To feel more confident, improve my health, and reduce stress on my joints."

Step 2: Decide which stress-management techniques you will incorporate into your daily routine. When you feel stressed, it could be 10 minutes of morning meditation or deep breathing techniques.

Step 3: If you choose not to follow the suggested meal plan, review the list of hormone-balancing foods and nutrients, and mark off the foods you already consume on a regular basis. Start adding in others that address the specific symptoms you are experiencing.

Suppose you decide to follow the meal plan in this book. In that case, you can still add other items from the lists that you'd like to eat more to alleviate specific negative symptoms.

It's recommended to keep a food journal when adding in new foods. Add only 1 or 2 at a time and note how you feel. This will help pinpoint any food sensitivities, food triggers, or any foods that provide relief.

Step 4: Incorporate a consistent exercise routine. Just 4 to 5 workout sessions a week of 30-45 minutes each will be plenty. Remember that excessive exercise can be perceived by your body as stress... so don't overdo it. Aim for 3-4 quality cardio sessions, and at least 2 strength training sessions, including free weights and machines for variety. You need at least one rest day a week, and adding a day for flexibility/mobility is a great practice.

Remember, the benefits of strength training include increased testosterone production, which helps burn fat and improve libido.

Step 5: Optimize your sleep. Aim for 7 to 8 hours each night. Pick one or two sleep-improving techniques and create a nightly routine to make this possible.

It may take some trial and error, depending on how off your sleep cycles are. Keeping a journal for this could be helpful as well as your work to find what works for your body.

Remember there is nothing wrong with testing a natural sleep aid. Speak to your healthcare provider before trying any supplements recommended.

Step 6: Stay hydrated. Drink at least half your body weight in ounces of water per day. If you are exercising you should get a bit more.

Note: Opt for a stainless steel or glass water bottle. Plastic water bottles contain BPAs, which can disrupt the endocrine system and throw your hormones off balance, making it harder to lose weight.

If you want to take your hormone balance a step further, join my Hormone Hacking for Weight Loss program. I go deeper into toxins and walk you through a simple elimination process to take your results to the next level.

Step 7: Get some social support by joining a group fitness class or our FREE online community to help you stay motivated and accountable.

www.facebook.com/groups/hormonehackingandnaturalfatloss

Step 8: Track your progress. That goes for your weight and your non-scale victories... they all count and improve your chances of sticking it out and reaching your goals.

I recommend weighing yourself weekly or biweekly on the same morning—before you eat or drink anything and after you've relieved your bladder and/or bowels. This is when it will be its most accurate using a scale.

Also pay attention to how your clothes fit, how you feel, your energy, confidence, and sleep. These are non-scale victories and can often be more rewarding than just the weight.

I have provided an example goal sheet/checklist to help you create your own and a blank one you can fill out for yourself in your bonuses.

Download it at:
hackyourhormonesforweightloss/bonuses

And remember you've got this!!!
Yours Truly, Hormone.Hacker
#aginglongevity

28-Day Meal Plan and Recipes

These hormone weight-loss meal plans and recipes boost your metabolism. They also take out the guesswork. You won't have to worry about what to eat—so refreshing. For me, the best part is knowing exactly what I'm eating every single day... not to have to think about it means one less decision I have to make today. There's no question. When the meals are there and the plan is done, you won't fall victim to all the fast-food tomfoolery out there.

These are dietitian-approved suggested meal plans and the rule of thumb is if you want to swap something out, swap "like for like." For example: If you don't like the suggested fish or chicken, swap it for another lean white meat. The same goes for carbs (starch for starch), non-starchy veggie or fruit for non-starchy veggie or fruit.

My clients have lost an average of 8-10 pounds on this 28-day plan. Imagine trimming an inch or two off of your waist... imagine being 8-10 pounds lighter next month!

Stop hiding from those holiday pictures. Be ready for the new year—without skipping Christmas. You'll have a head start on those New Year's resolutions and you'll be ahead of the game, already working on your next goal!

Be your best with these nourishing, hormone-balancing meals.

Breakfast

- Arugula and Eggs
- Blackberry Apple Smoothie
- Blueberry Macadamia Breakfast Cookies
- Coconut Mango Oat Milk Oatmeal
- Cottage Cheese Bowl
- Green Glow Smoothie
- Mango Smoothie Bowl
- Sweet Potato Pear Smoothie Bowl
- Turkey Breakfast Hash
- Zucchini Tahini Muffins

Lunch

- Beef and Rice Bowl
- Bunless "Greek" Burger
- Eggs and Greens
- Grab 'n' Go Lunch
- Green Goddess Salad
- Ground Turkey Lettuce Wraps
- Pulled Chicken Wrap
- Simple Salad
- Summer Salad
- Thai-Inspired Quinoa Salad

Dinner
- Buttery Chicken Sheet Pan Dinner
- Fried Quinoa
- Garlic Basil Pasta
- Parsley Salmon with Vegetable Quinoa
- Pork Roast with Cauliflower and Sweet Potato
- Roasted Chicken Thighs with Sweet Potato & Broccoli
- Roasted Potatoes and Carrots with Chicken
- Sautéed Brussels Sprouts and Chicken
- Shrimp Asparagus Pasta
- Traditional Steak & Potatoes

WEEK 1

Sunday

B Blueberry Macadamia Breakfast Cookies *(freeze remaining)*

L Pulled Chicken Wrap

D Garlic Basil Pasta

Monday

B Arugula and Eggs

L Beef and Rice Bowl *(freeze leftovers for tomorrow)*

D Garlic Basil Pasta

Tuesday

B Blackberry Apple Smoothie

L Beef and Rice Bowl

D Sautéed Brussels Sprouts and Chicken

Wednesday

B Arugula and Eggs

L Simple Salad

D Sautéed Brussels Sprouts and Chicken

Thursday

B Blackberry Apple Smoothie

L Simple Salad

D Pork Roast with Cauliflower and Sweet Potato

Friday

B Blueberry Macadamia Breakfast Cookies

L Bunless "Greek" Burger

D Pork Roast with Cauliflower and Sweet Potato

Saturday

B Cottage Cheese Bowl

L Bunless "Greek" Burger

D Fried Quinoa

Week 1 Shopping List

Produce

2 stalks celery
2 small red onions
3 bulbs garlic
6 cups arugula
2 yellow onions
4 medium scallions/green
  onions
3 cups Brussels sprouts
2 heads cauliflower
4 sweet potatoes
1 cucumber

1 small head cabbage
  (or shredded cabbage)
1 cup grapes
1 cup shredded carrots
1/2 cup blueberries
1 1/4 cup blackberries
1 cantaloupe
5-6 apples
1 bundle fresh dill
1 bundle fresh basil
1 bundle fresh rosemary
1 cup broccoli sprouts

Meat/Poultry/Dairy

7 eggs
1 oz mozzarella cheese
1 cup 4% milk fat cottage
  cheese
1 jar ghee
6 oz ground turkey

5 chicken breasts
12 oz ground beef
  (95% lean)
8 oz pork tenderloin
10 oz ground lamb

Grains/Beans/Nuts/Legumes

1/4 cup macadamia nuts
1/2 cup almond flour
Small container coconut
  flour

4 1/2 tbsp chia seeds
Small container flax seed
Small container hemp
  hearts or seeds

Miscellaneous

Oat milk
Almond milk
Ground oregano

Coconut aminos
Cassava flour
6 oz brown rice pasta

Week 1 Meal Prep

For dinner meals Sunday through Thursday, freeze the second portion to be warmed for dinner the following evening.

Sunday evening, cook the following and store in the freezer:

> Beef and rice bowl, for lunches on Monday and Tuesday.

> Two chicken breasts, for salad at lunches on Wednesday and Thursday.

> Two lamb burgers from the bunless "Greek" burger recipe, for lunches on Friday and Saturday.

Wednesday and Thursday morning, remove a chicken breast from the freezer to thaw. Prepare lunch salad separately.

Friday and Saturday morning, remove lamb burgers from the freezer to thaw. Prepare sauce and vegetables for lunch separately.

DAILY AVERAGES

CALORIES: 1,436
CARBOHYDRATES: 128 G   PROTEIN: 82 G   FAT: 70 G

WEEK 2

Sunday
B Turkey Breakfast Hash *(freeze remaining)*

L Simple Salad

D Traditional Steak & Potatoes *(make 1/2 recipe)*

Monday
B Zucchini Tahini Muffins *(freeze remaining)*

L Ground Turkey Lettuce Wraps

D Traditional Steak & Potatoes *(make 1/2 recipe)*

Tuesday
B Coconut Mango Oat Milk Oatmeal

L Ground Turkey Lettuce Wraps

D Roasted Chicken Thighs with Sweet Potato & Broccoli

Wednesday
B Zucchini Tahini Muffins

L Grab 'n' Go Lunch

D Roasted Chicken Thighs with Sweet Potato & Broccoli

Thursday
B Coconut Mango Oat Milk Oatmeal

L Grab 'n' Go Lunch

D Buttery Chicken Sheet Pan Dinner

Friday
B Turkey Breakfast Hash

L Green Goddess Salad *(save 1/2 for tomorrow, dressing separately)*

D Buttery Chicken Sheet Pan Dinner

Saturday
B Arugula and Eggs

L Green Goddess Salad

D Parsley Salmon with Vegetable Quinoa

Week 2 Shopping List

Produce

4-5 sweet potatoes
3 cups Brussels sprouts
3 cups arugula
1/2 cup kale
1 red onion
1 yellow onion
2 russet potatoes
1 zucchini
1 bulb garlic
1 red bell pepper
1 head romaine lettuce
2 heads broccoli
6 oz baby potatoes
1 head red cabbage

6 radishes
1 cucumber
3 scallions/green onions
4 cups mixed salad greens,
    without spinach
1 bundle fresh parsley
1 bundle chives
1 bundle fresh dill
1 bundle fresh mint
1 red apple
1 green apple
2 mangos
2 cups grapes
1 cantaloupe

Meat/Poultry/Dairy

9 eggs
1 small jar ghee
3/4 lb turkey breast

3 chicken breasts
12 oz ground turkey

Grains/Beans/Nuts/Legumes

1/4 cup pecans
Small container flax seed
Small jar tahini
1 1/4 tbsp sesame seeds
Small jar almond butter
1 1/2 cup rolled oats

1/4 cup quinoa
1/2 cup macadamia nuts
2/3 cup sunflower seeds
Small container hemp
    hearts or seeds
1/2 cup pumpkin seeds

Miscellaneous

Oat milk (or substitute
with almond milk)
Almond milk
1/4 cup coconut cream
Cassava flour
Arrowroot flour
Garlic powder
Ground turmeric
Ground ginger
Onion powder

Dried oregano
Dried thyme
Olive oil
Avocado oil
Honey
Salt & Pepper
2 tbsp coconut flakes
Baking powder
Baking soda
Coconut sugar

Week 2 Meal Prep

For dinner meals on Tuesday and Thursday, freeze second portion to be warmed for dinner the following evening.

Freeze half recipe of turkey breakfast hash for breakfast on Friday.

Sunday evening, cook ground turkey mixture for lettuce wraps Monday and Tuesday. Remove from freezer to thaw on Monday and Tuesday morning.

Sunday evening, cook zucchini tahini muffins and store them in the freezer. Warm in microwave when ready to eat. These will be had again in week 4.

Wednesday morning and Thursday morning, make three hard-boiled eggs to be had with lunch.

Saturday morning, remove salmon from the freezer to defrost before making for dinner that evening.

DAILY AVERAGES

CALORIES: 1,416
CARBOHYDRATES: 116 G   PROTEIN: 83 G   FAT: 73 G

WEEK 3

Sunday
B Green Glow Smoothie
L Bunless "Greek" Burger
D Roasted Potatoes and Carrots with Chicken

Monday
B Sweet Potato Pear Smoothie Bowl
L Thai-Inspired Quinoa Salad
D Roasted Potatoes and Carrots with Chicken

Tuesday
B Turkey Breakfast Hash *(freeze second portion)*
L Thai-Inspired Quinoa Salad
D Traditional Steak & Potatoes *(make 1/2 recipe)*

Wednesday
B Sweet Potato Pear Smoothie Bowl
L Summer Salad
D Traditional Steak & Potatoes *(make 1/2 recipe)*

Thursday
B Turkey Breakfast Hash
L Summer Salad
D Garlic Basil Pasta

Friday
B Green Glow Smoothie
L Pulled Chicken Wrap
D Garlic Basil Pasta

Saturday
B Arugula and Eggs
L Pulled Chicken Wrap
D Shrimp Asparagus Pasta

Week 3 Shopping List

Produce

3 cups baby kale
5 cups arugula
2 bulbs garlic
1 cucumber
1 red onion
1 yellow onion
8 carrots
1 small head red cabbage
1 med scallion/red onion
1 cup sugar snap peas
4 sweet potatoes
3 cups Brussels sprouts
2 russet potatoes
4 celery stalks

1 small bundle asparagus
1 bundle chives
1 bundle fresh dill
1 bundle fresh cilantro
1 bundle fresh mint
1 bundle fresh basil
1 bundle fresh parsley
1 mango
2 green apples
2 pears
1/2 cup blueberries
2 cups grapes
1 cantaloupe
1 1/2 lbs baby potatoes

Meat/Poultry/Dairy

1 cup 2% cottage cheese
6 oz mozzarella cheese
3 eggs

1 small jar ghee
4 chic drumsticks, skin on
12 oz ribeye steak

Grains/Beans/Nuts/Legumes

Small container flax seed
Small container hemp
  hearts or seeds
1/2 cup sunflower seeds

Small jar sunflower seed
  butter
1/2 cup macadamia nuts
1 cup quinoa
9 oz brown rice pasta

Miscellaneous

Dried oregano
Dried ginger
Garlic powder

Coconut aminos
Almond milk
  (cont'd on next page)

1/2 container coconut
 yogurt
Olive oil
Avocado oil
Sesame oil
Honey
Cassava flour tortillas

Week 3 Meal Prep

For dinner meals on Sunday and Thursday, freeze the second portion to be warmed for dinner the following evening.

On Sunday:

> Boil two sweet potatoes. Cool, peel, and freeze for Sweet Potato Pear Smoothie Bowl to be had on Monday and Tuesday.

> Cook quinoa and store in freezer (portions stored separately) for Thai-Inspired Quinoa Salad on Monday and Tuesday. Remove from freezer on Monday and Tuesday morning.

> Option to cook Turkey Breakfast Hash ahead of time and store in freezer, to be had for breakfast on Tuesday and Thursday.

Thursday evening, make two chicken breasts to be had with lunch on Friday and Saturday. Store in freezer and remove the morning of.

Thaw shrimp under cool water just before cooking dinner on Saturday.

DAILY AVERAGES

CALORIES: 1,492
CARBOHYDRATES: 135 G   PROTEIN: 81 G   FAT: 72 G

WEEK 4

Sunday
B Mango Smoothie Bowl
L Thai-Inspired Quinoa Salad
D Roasted Chicken Thighs with Sweet Potato and Broccoli

Monday
B Zucchini Tahini Muffins
L Ground Turkey Lettuce Wraps
D Roasted Chicken Thighs with Sweet Potato and Broccoli

Tuesday
B Cottage Cheese Bowl
L Ground Turkey Lettuce Wraps
D Traditional Steak & Potatoes

Wednesday
B Zucchini Tahini Muffins
L Eggs and Greens
D Traditional Steak & Potatoes

Thursday
B Cottage Cheese Bowl
L Eggs and Greens
D Roasted Potatoes and Carrots with Chicken

Friday
B Mango Smoothie Bowl
L Summer Salad
D Roasted Potatoes and Carrots with Chicken

Saturday
B Arugula and Eggs
L Summer Salad
D Parsley Salmon with Vegetable Quinoa

Week 4 Shopping List

Produce

1 small head red cabbage
8 carrots
5 scallions/green onions
1/2 cup sugar snap peas
2 heads broccoli
2 sweet potatoes
2 zucchinis
1 large bulb garlic
1 red bell pepper
1 medium yellow onion
1/2 cup kale
1 large cucumber
2 russet potatoes
1/2 cup raspberries
1/2 cup blueberries

2 medium peaches
1/2 cup blackberries
2 tbsp fresh chives
1 bundle fresh dill
1 bundle fresh mint
1 bundle fresh cilantro
5 cups arugula or rocket
4 cups mixed salad greens
   without spinach
1 bundle fresh parsley
1 bundle romaine lettuce
2 cups frozen mango
1/4 cup apple sauce
1 cantaloupe
1 1/2 lbs baby potatoes

Meat/Poultry/Dairy

2 cups 2% milk-fat cottage
   cheese
1/4 cup ricotta cheese
4 oz mozzarella cheese
1 jar ghee
6 oz frozen salmon
12 oz ribeye steak

7 eggs
8 oz chicken thighs,
   boneless and skinless
12 oz ground turkey
4 chicken drumsticks,
   skin on

Grains/Beans/Nuts/Legumes

1 cup sunflower seeds
2 tbsp chia seeds
Small jar sunflower seed
   butter
Small jar almond butter

Small jar tahini
Small container flax seed
3/4 cup quinoa
1/4 cup walnuts
1/2 cup macadamia nuts

1/4 cup almond milk
Oat milk (or substitute
    with almond milk)

1 1/4 tbsp sesame seeds
7 tbsp hemp hearts or
    seeds

Miscellaneous

Cassava flour
Arrowroot flour
Stevia
Ground ginger
Garlic powder
Ground turmeric
Dried oregano

Salt
Pepper
Coconut aminos
Baking powder
Sesame oil
Olive oil
Avocado oil

Week 4 Meal Prep

For dinner meals on Sunday and Thursday, freeze the second portion to be warmed for dinner the following evening.

If you do not have leftover Zucchini Tahini Muffins in the freezer from week 2, bake these muffins on Sunday and store in the freezer until ready to warm up in the microwave.

Sunday evening, cook ground turkey mixture to be had with lettuce wraps for lunch on Monday and Tuesday. Remove from freezer to thaw on Monday and Tuesday morning.

Wednesday morning and Thursday morning make two hard-boiled eggs to be had with lunch.

Saturday morning remove salmon from the freezer to defrost before making for dinner that evening.

DAILY AVERAGES

CALORIES: 1,433
CARBOHYDRATES: 104 G   PROTEIN: 77 G   FAT: 81 G

BREAKFAST

ARUGULA AND EGGS

SERVINGS: 1   PREP TIME: 5 MIN.   COOKING TIME: 5 MIN.

Ingredients

1 tsp ghee
1/4 cup yellow onion, chopped
3 large eggs, beaten
Himalayan salt and pepper, to taste
1 cup arugula or rocket
1 tbsp hemp seeds
1 1/2 cups cantaloupe, chopped

Directions

1.   Warm ghee in medium skillet over medium heat.

2.   Add onion and cook 2-3 minutes

3.   Add eggs, salt, and pepper. Cook approximately 1 minute, scraping from the pan with a soft spatula as it cooks.

4.   Add arugula or rocket and continue as above, until eggs are desired consistency.

5.   Top with hemp seeds and serve with cantaloupe.

CALORIES: 411, CARBOHYDRATE 24 GR, PROTEIN: 26 GR, FAT: 24 GR

BLACKBERRY APPLE SMOOTHIE

SERVINGS: 1   PREP TIME: 5 MIN.   COOKING TIME: 0 MIN.

Ingredients

2 tbsp chia seeds
1 tbsp ground flaxseed
1/2 cup blackberries
1 medium size apple (cored)
1/8 cup oats
1 cup oat milk
1/4 cup water
1/2 cup ice

Directions

1. Combine all ingredients in a blender and blend until smooth.

2. Serve cold and enjoy!

CALORIES: 495, CARBOHYDRATE 73 GR, PROTEIN: 13 GR, FAT: 19 GR

BLUEBERRY MACADAMIA BREAKFAST COOKIES

SERVINGS: 4   PREP TIME: 10 MIN. COOKING TIME: 10-12 MIN.

Ingredients

1/4 cup Macadamia nuts, chopped
1 cup almond flour
1/3 cup coconut flour
2 tbsp honey
2 large eggs, beaten
1/3 cup almond milk
1 tbsp ghee, melted
1/2 cup blueberries

Directions

1. Preheat oven to 325 degrees F.

2. Mix all ingredients together, except for blueberries, until well blended. Lightly mix in blueberries.

3. Make 8 balls with the dough and lightly press onto a cookie tray.

4. Cook for 10-12 minutes, until lightly browned.

CALORIES: 392, CARBOHYDRATE 24 GR, PROTEIN: 14 GR, FAT: 28 GR

COCONUT MANGO OAT MILK OATMEAL

SERVINGS: 2   PREP TIME: 5 MIN.   COOKING TIME: 15 MIN.

Ingredients

1/2 cup oat milk
1/2 cup water
3/4 cup dry rolled oats
Dash of salt
3/4 cup mango
1 tbsp coconut flakes, unsweetened
1 tbsp hemp hearts

Directions

1. Combine the oat milk, water, dry rolled oats, salt, and stevia in a saucepan.

2. Bring to a boil and, once boiling, simmer for 10-12 minutes or until the oats are cooked and the oat milk and water is fully absorbed.

3. While the oats are cooking, chop the mango into small pieces.

4. Remove the cooked oats from the pan and serve in a bowl.

5. Top with mango and coconut. Serve warm and enjoy!

CALORIES: 446, CARBOHYDRATE 73 GR, PROTEIN: 13 GR, FAT: 14 GR

COTTAGE CHEESE BOWL

SERVINGS: 1   PREP TIME: 2 MIN.   COOKING TIME: 0 MIN.

Ingredients

1 cup 4% milk fat cottage cheese, organic
1/4 cup blueberries
1/4 cup blackberries
1/2 tbsp chia seeds
1 tbsp pecans, chopped

Directions

1.   Top cottage cheese with all other ingredients.

CALORIES: 335, CARBOHYDRATE 22 GR, PROTEIN: 28 GR, FAT: 16 GR

GREEN GLOW SMOOTHIE

SERVINGS: 1   PREP TIME: 5 MIN.   COOKING TIME: 0 MIN.

Ingredients

1/2 cup kale, chopped
1 tbsp flaxseed
1/2 cup 4% milk fat cottage cheese, organic
1/2 cup frozen mango
1 medium apple, sliced
1 cup almond milk

Directions

1.   Blend all ingredients together in a blender and enjoy!

CALORIES: 371, CARBOHYDRATE 48 GR, PROTEIN: 17 GR, FAT: 13 GR

MANGO SMOOTHIE BOWL

SERVINGS: 1   PREP TIME: 5 MIN.   COOKING TIME: 0 MIN.

Ingredients

2 cups of frozen mango
1/2 cup oat milk
1/4 tsp stevia
1 tbsp hemp seeds
1 1/2 tbsp sunflower seeds
1 tbsp chia seeds

Directions

1. Combine the frozen mango, oat milk, stevia, and hemp seeds in a blender.

2. Pour into a bowl and top with sunflower seeds and chia seeds.

CALORIES: 384, CARBOHYDRATE 46 GR, PROTEIN: 11 GR, FAT: 19 GR

SWEET POTATO PEAR SMOOTHIE BOWL

SERVINGS: 1   PREP TIME: 5 MIN.   COOKING TIME: 0 MIN.

Ingredients

1 cup unsweetened non-dairy milk of choice
1 med Japanese or white sweet potato, cooked,
   peeled and frozen
1 medium pear, cored, and diced
2 handfuls baby spinach
2 tbsp hemp hearts
1/4 tsp ground ginger

Directions

Blend all ingredients together in a blender until smooth. Enjoy!

CALORIES: 402, CARBOHYDRATE 65 GR, PROTEIN: 12 GR, FAT: 12 GR

TURKEY BREAKFAST HASH

SERVINGS: 2   PREP TIME: 10 MIN. COOKING TIME: 30-40 MIN.

Ingredients

3/4 lb turkey breast
1 tbsp fresh dill, chopped
1/2 tbsp garlic powder
1 tbsp ghee
2 medium sweet potatoes
3 cups Brussels sprouts
Salt and pepper, to taste

Directions

1. Preheat the oven to 350 degrees F.

2. Season the turkey breast with garlic powder, dill, salt and pepper.

3. Bake 12 -20 minutes until internal temperature reaches 165 degrees F.

4. While the turkey is cooking, heat a sauté pan on medium heat and melt the ghee in the pan.

5. Chop the sweet potato into half-inch cubes/pieces and chop the brussels sprouts into halves.

6. Sauté the sweet potatoes, Brussels sprouts, and salt and pepper in the ghee for 10-12 minutes or until the sweet potatoes are cooked and the Brussels sprouts are crispy.

7. Slice the turkey breast on top of the hash.

8. Serve warm and enjoy!

CALORIES: 450, CARBOHYDRATE 40 GR, PROTEIN: 47 GR, FAT: 12 GR

ZUCCHINI TAHINI MUFFINS

SERVINGS: 8   PREP TIME: 10 MIN.   COOKING TIME: 25 MIN.

Ingredients

1 tbsp ground flaxseed
2.5 tbsp water
1/2 cup tahini
1/3 cup coconut sugar
3 tbsp unsweetened non-dairy milk of choice
3 tbsp unsweetened applesauce
1 cup finely shredded zucchini
1 cup cassava flour
1/4 cup arrowroot flour
1 tsp baking powder
1/2 tsp baking soda
1/4 tsp fine sea salt
sesame seeds for sprinkling (optional)
4 tbsp almond butter

Directions

1. Preheat oven to 350 degrees F. Coat a muffin pan with cooking oil or use silicone liners.

2. Combine the flaxseed and water together in a large bowl. Whisk and let sit for 5-10 minutes until thick and gel-like.

3. Whisk in the tahini, coconut sugar, applesauce, and milk. Stir in the grated zucchini.

4. Mix in dry ingredients until just combined.

5. Scoop batter into muffin cups, filling each one almost to the top. Sprinkle tops with sesame seeds if desired.

6. Bake for 22-25 minutes or until a toothpick inserted into the center comes out clean.

7. Allow to cool 10 minutes before transferring to a wire rack.

8.   Spread with almond butter before serving.

CALORIES: 426, CARBOHYDRATE 51 GR, PROTEIN: 8 GR, FAT: 23 GR

LUNCH

BEEF AND RICE BOWL

SERVINGS: 2   PREP TIME: 5 MIN.   COOKING TIME: 20 MIN.

Ingredients

3/4 cup white rice
3/4 lb ground beef (95% lean)
Salt and pepper to taste
4 stalks green onion, chopped
1 cup broccoli sprouts

Directions

1. Cook rice as directed on package.

2. Add ground beef, salt, and pepper to a medium skillet and cook over medium heat for 4-6 minutes, until browned through, crumbling as you cook.

3. Top rice with ground beef, green onion, and broccoli sprouts.

CALORIES: 496, CARBOHYDRATE 59 GR, PROTEIN: 43 GR, FAT: 9 GR

Bunless "Greek" Burger

SERVINGS: 2   PREP TIME: 10-15 MIN.   COOKING TIME: 10 MIN.

Ingredients

For Burger:

10 oz ground lamb
1/2 small red onion (chop half, slice half)
1 tbsp oregano
1 tbsp minced garlic
salt and pepper to taste
1 tbsp olive oil
1/4 of a small cucumber

For Homemade Tzatziki:

1 container (5 oz) coconut yogurt
1/4 cup thinly sliced cucumber
1 tsp olive oil
1 tbsp dill
1/2 tbsp garlic (chopped/minced)
Salt and pepper to taste

Directions

1. Combine ground lamb, 1/4 cup chopped red onion, oregano, minced garlic, salt and pepper in a bowl.

2. Once combined, form into two patties.

3. Over medium-high heat, heat olive oil in a skillet.

4. Once the skillet and oil are hot, place the lamb patties on the skillet.

5. Let it cook for 3-4 minutes, then flip.

6. Cook until the patties reach 160 degrees F and remove from the skillet to rest.

7. While the patties are cooking, slice the remaining red onion and cucumber for the toppings.

8. For the tzatziki, combine coconut yogurt, sliced cucumber, olive oil, dill, and garlic in a small bowl.

9. Plate the burger and top with cucumber, red onion, and a dollop of homemade tzatziki. Enjoy!

CALORIES: 584, CARBOHYDRATE 11 GR, PROTEIN: 30 GR, FAT: 47 GR

EGGS AND GREENS

SERVINGS: 1   PREP TIME: 10 MIN.   COOKING TIME: 10 MIN.

Ingredients

2 eggs
2 cups mixed salad greens (without spinach)
1 tbsp hemp hearts
2 stalks green onion
1 peach, chopped
1 tsp dried oregano
2 tbsp ricotta cheese
1 tbsp olive oil
Salt and pepper to taste

Directions

1. Hard boil two eggs in boiling water for 10 minutes. Allow to cool. Peel and cut in half.

2. Top salad greens with all other ingredients and enjoy!

CALORIES: 447, CARBOHYDRATE 24 GR, PROTEIN: 22 GR, FAT: 31 GR

GRAB 'N' GO LUNCH

SERVINGS: 1   PREP TIME: 2 MIN.   COOKING TIME: 0 MIN.

Ingredients

3 hard-boiled eggs
1/4 cup macadamia nuts
1 cup purple grapes

Directions

1.   Pack all together and go!

CALORIES: 555, CARBOHYDRATE 23 GR, PROTEIN: 22 GR, FAT: 40 GR

GREEN GODDESS SALAD

SERVINGS: 2   PREP TIME: 10 MIN.   COOKING TIME: 0 MIN.

Ingredients

Salad Mix:

4 cups mixed salad greens (without spinach)
6 medium radishes (chopped)
1 medium cucumber (chopped)
1 green apple, chopped
3 stalks green onion, chopped
3 tbsp sunflower seeds
2 tbsp hemp hearts
2 tbsp pumpkin seeds

Dressing:

1 1/2 tbsp coconut cream (top layer in canned coconut milk)
2 tbsp olive oil
1/4 cup fresh dill
1/4 cup fresh mint
Salt and pepper to taste

Directions

1. In a blender, blend all dressing ingredients together until smooth.

2. Toss all salad ingredients together with dressing until well coated and enjoy!

CALORIES: 435, CARBOHYDRATE 31 GR, PROTEIN: 12 GR, FAT: 32 GR

GROUND TURKEY LETTUCE WRAPS

SERVINGS: 2 PREP TIME: 10 MIN. COOKING TIME: 5-7 MIN.

Ingredients

3/4 lb ground turkey
1 tbsp avocado oil
3 cloves garlic, minced or pressed
1/4 tsp ground turmeric
1/4 tbsp ground ginger
Salt and pepper to taste
1 red bell pepper, chopped
1 small yellow onion, chopped
1 tbsp sesame seeds

Dressing:

2 tbsp tahini
1 tbsp honey
1/2 tbsp water
1 head bibb lettuce

Directions

1. Heat avocado oil over medium heat in a large skillet. Add garlic, turkey, turmeric, and ginger. Cook for approximately 3-4minutes until lightly pink, crumbling and flipping as it cooks.

2. Add salt, pepper, red bell pepper, onion, and sesame seeds. Cook for an additional 2-3 minutes. Remove from heat.

3. Mix together tahini, honey, and water in a blender and blend until smooth.

4. Separate, wash, and pat dry bib lettuce leaves. Top leaves with turkey mixture and tahini dressing. Enjoy!

CALORIES: 489, CARBOHYDRATE 22 GR, PROTEIN: 38 GR, FAT: 29 GR

PULLED CHICKEN WRAP

SERVINGS: 1   PREP TIME: 15 MIN.   COOKING TIME: 25 MIN.

Ingredients

1 chicken breast
1/4 tbsp avocado oil
Salt and pepper to taste
1 cassava flour wrap
1 stalk celery
1/2 tbsp olive oil
1/4 small red onion, chopped
1/2 tbsp dried dill
Salt and pepper to taste
1 oz mozzarella cheese, chopped
1/2 cup grapes

Directions

1. Preheat oven to 375 degrees F. Brush chicken breast with oil and sprinkle with salt and pepper. Bake for approximately 25 minutes in an oven-safe dish, until internal temperature of chicken breast reaches 165 degrees F.

2. Using a fork, shred chicken and allow to cool. Mix chicken with celery, olive oil, red onion, dill, salt, and pepper.

3. Fill cassava flour tortilla with shredded chicken mixture and mozzarella. Fold over and serve with a side of grapes.

CALORIES: 502, CARBOHYDRATE 45 GR, PROTEIN: 35 GR, FAT: 21 GR

SIMPLE SALAD

SERVINGS: 1   PREP TIME: 5 MIN.   COOKING TIME: 25 MIN.

Ingredients

2 cups arugula or rocket
1 medium red or green apple, sliced
2 tbsp chopped pecans
1/4 small red onion, chopped
1 chicken breast
1 tbsp olive oil
Salt and pepper to taste

Directions

1. Preheat oven to 400 degrees F. Bake chicken breast after brushing with olive oil, salt and pepper for approximately 25 minutes; slice into 1/2 inch slices when cooled.

2. Add arugula, apple, pecans, red onion, and sliced chicken breast to a salad bowl. Toss with olive oil, salt, and pepper.

3. Enjoy!

CALORIES: 467, CARBOHYDRATE 30 GR, PROTEIN: 30 GR, FAT: 27 GR

SUMMER SALAD

SERVINGS: 1   PREP TIME: 10 MIN.   COOKING TIME: 0 MIN.

Ingredients

2 cups arugula
1/2 medium cucumber, chopped
1/4 cup blueberries
1/4 cup macadamia nuts, chopped
2 oz mozzarella cheese
2 tbsp fresh dill, chopped
1 tbsp fresh mint, chopped
1 tbsp olive oil
Salt and pepper to taste

Directions

1. Toss together all ingredients in a large salad bowl and
    enjoy!

CALORIES: 574, CARBOHYDRATE 15 GR, PROTEIN: 17 GR, FAT: 52 GR

THAI-INSPIRED QUINOA SALAD

SERVINGS: 2   PREP TIME: 10 MIN.   COOKING TIME: 0 MIN.

Ingredients

Salad:

1 cup cooked quinoa
1 cup shredded red cabbage
1/2 cup shredded carrots
3/4 cup sugar snap peas
1/4 cup chopped cilantro
2 tbsp chopped green onion
2 tbsp roasted sunflower seeds

Dressing:

1/4 cup unsweetened sunflower butter
1/2 tbsp coconut aminos
1 tbsp toasted sesame oil
1/2 tbsp freshly grated ginger
Water for desired consistency

Directions

1. In a large bowl, combine the cooked quinoa, red cabbage, carrots, sugar snap peas, cilantro, and green onion. Set aside.

2. To make the dressing, whisk the sunflower butter, lime juice, coconut aminos, sesame oil, and ginger in a small bowl. Mix in a tablespoon of water at a time to reach desired consistency.

3. Pour the dressing into the salad and toss well to combine.

4. Divide into individual servings and top with roasted sunflower seeds.

CALORIES: 464, CARBOHYDRATE 38 GR, PROTEIN: 13 GR, FAT: 31 GR

Dinner

Buttery Chicken Sheet Pan Dinner

SERVINGS: 2   PREP TIME: 10 MIN. COOKING TIME: 20-25 MIN.

Ingredients

3 tbsp ghee, melted
1 small head of purple cabbage, sliced into 1/2 inch circles
6 oz baby potatoes
2, 5oz chicken breasts, pounded to tenderize
1/2 tbsp dried oregano
1 tsp garlic powder
1 tsp onion powder
1 tsp dried thyme
Himalayan salt and pepper to taste

Directions

1.   Preheat oven to 425 degrees F.

2.   In a small bowl mix together oregano, garlic powder, onion powder, thyme, salt, and pepper.

3.   Spread cabbage, potatoes, and chicken on an oven-safe pan. Coat with melted ghee and seasoning mix.

4.   Bake in the oven for 20-25 minutes until internal temperature of chicken reaches 165 degrees F.

5.   Remove from the oven and allow 5 minutes to rest before eating.

CALORIES: 488, CARBOHYDRATE 38 GR, PROTEIN: 33 GR, FAT: 25 GR

FRIED QUINOA

SERVINGS: 2   PREP TIME: 10 MIN.   COOKING TIME: 20 MIN.

Ingredients

3/4 cup quinoa, uncooked
1 tbsp ghee
3 cloves garlic, minced
1/4 cup slivered almonds
1 small onion, chopped
4 cups shredded cabbage
2 cups carrots, shredded
1 1/2 tbsp coconut aminos
Pepper to taste

Directions

1. Cook quinoa as directed on package.
2. Melt ghee in a large skillet over medium heat. Add almonds and garlic and cook 1-2 minutes until fragrant.
3. Add onions to the skillet and cook 1 additional minute.
4. Add the cabbage and carrots to the skillet and cook until soft, or desired consistency (approximately 5 minutes).
5. Lastly, add cooked quinoa, coconut aminos, and pepper and cook 2-3minutes.
6. Serve warm.

CALORIES: 519, CARBOHYDRATE 77 GR, PROTEIN: 17 GR, FAT: 18 GR

GARLIC BASIC PASTA

SERVINGS: 2   PREP TIME: 5 MIN. COOKING TIME: 20-25 MIN.

Ingredients

6 oz dry brown rice pasta
6 oz ground turkey
1 1/2 tbsp ghee, divided
2 tbsp chopped garlic
1/4 cup chopped basil
Salt and pepper to taste

Directions

1. Cook the pasta per the directions on the package and set aside.

2. In a sauté pan, heat ghee over medium heat.

3. Once hot, add the chopped garlic and sauté until golden brown. Add turkey and cook 5-8minutes, crumbling and turning as you go along.

4. Add the basil.

5. Season with salt and pepper.

6. Add the pasta back into the butter garlic, turkey, basil sauce.

7. Serve warm and enjoy!

CALORIES: 545, CARBOHYDRATE 67 GR, PROTEIN: 25 GR, FAT: 20 GR

PARSLEY SALMON WITH VEGETABLE QUINOA

SERVINGS: 2   PREP TIME: 10 MIN.   COOKING TIME: 30-40 MIN.

Ingredients

2, 6oz wild salmon filets
1/2 tbsp garlic powder
2 tbsp fresh chopped parsley
Salt and pepper to taste
1 tbsp ghee
1/2 cup quinoa, uncooked
1 cup zucchini, sliced thin
1 cup kale, chopped
1 tbsp chopped/minced garlic

Directions

1. Cook the quinoa per the directions on the packaging and set aside.

2. In a sauté pan, heat 1 tbsp ghee over medium heat.

3. While the pan is heating up, season the salmon with garlic powder, salt, pepper, and fresh chopped parsley.

4. Place the fish in the sauté pan, cook to desired temperature and set aside.

5. In the same sauté pan, over medium heat, sauté zucchini, kale, and black beans for 4-5 minutes or until the zucchini begins to brown and the kale turns bright green.

6. Mix the quinoa into vegetable mix in the pan.

7. Serve the salmon over the vegetable quinoa mix. Enjoy!

CALORIES: 461, CARBOHYDRATE 35 GR, PROTEIN: 43 GR, FAT: 17 GR

PORK ROAST
WITH CAULIFLOWER AND SWEET POTATO

SERVINGS: 2   PREP TIME: 15 MIN.   COOKING TIME: 25 MIN.

Ingredients

1/2 lb pork tenderloin
4 cups cauliflower florets
3 cups sweet potato, peeled and chopped into 1/2 inch pieces
2 tbsp avocado oil
4 cloves garlic, minced or pressed
1 tbsp fresh rosemary, chopped
Salt and pepper to taste
1/4 cup fresh parley, chopped

Directions

1. Preheat oven to 375 degrees F.

2. In a small bowl mix together avocado oil, garlic, rosemary, salt, and pepper.

3. Brush pork with avocado oil mixture and place on an oven-safe sheet pan.

4. Toss vegetables with remaining avocado oil mixture and spread onto the sheet pan in a single layer.

5. Cook pork and vegetables in the oven for approximately 25 minutes, until internal temperature reaches above 145 degrees F.

6. Slice pork into 1/2-inch slices and top meal with fresh parsley before serving.

CALORIES: 498, CARBOHYDRATE 54 GR, PROTEIN: 31 GR, FAT: 19 GR

ROASTED CHICKEN THIGHS WITH SWEET POTATO & BROCCOLI

SERVINGS: 2   PREP TIME: 10 MIN.   COOKING TIME: 30 MIN.

Ingredients

1 tbsp ghee
1.5 tbsp fresh dill
1/2 tbsp garlic powder
1/2 lb chicken thighs
2 cups sweet potato (chopped into 1/2 to 1-inch cubes)
2 cups broccoli
2 tbsp olive oil
Salt and pepper to taste

Directions

1. Preheat the oven to 375 degrees F.

2. In a small bowl, combine ghee, 1 tbsp of dill, garlic powder, salt and pepper. Stir until combined.

3. Lay chicken thighs on a non-stick, oven-safe baking sheet.

4. Spread the ghee/dill mixture evenly on the tops of the chicken thighs.

5. Place the broccoli and sweet potatoes in a bowl and drizzle with olive oil, salt, pepper, and 1/2 tbsp dill.

6. Spread the broccoli and sweet potatoes onto the baking sheet with the chicken.

7. Bake in the oven for 25-30 minutes or until the chicken is cooked to 165 F. Serve warm and enjoy!

CALORIES: 463, CARBOHYDRATE 35 GR, PROTEIN: 27 GR, FAT: 25 GR

ROASTED POTATOES AND CARROTS WITH CHICKEN

SERVINGS: 2   PREP TIME: 15 MIN.   COOKING TIME: 25 MIN.

Ingredients

8 medium carrots, peeled
4 cups baby potatoes, halved
2 tbsp avocado oil, divided
Salt and pepper to taste
4 chicken drumsticks, skin on
1 tbsp coconut aminos
1 tbsp honey
1/2 tsp dried ginger
1 tsp garlic powder

Directions

8. Preheat oven to 400 degrees F.

9. Spread carrots and potatoes onto a large cooking sheet and coat with 1 tbsp avocado oil, salt, and pepper to taste.

10. In a small bowl, mix together 1 tbsp avocado oil, coconut aminos, honey, ginger, and garlic.

11. Coat chicken drumsticks in coconut aminos mixture and add to the cooking sheet.

12. Bake for approximately 25 minutes, until internal temperature of chicken reaches 165 degrees F and potatoes are soft. Enjoy warm!

CALORIES: 658, CARBOHYDRATE 62 GR, PROTEIN: 34 GR, FAT: 28 GR

SAUTÉED BRUSSELS SPROUTS AND CHICKEN

SERVINGS: 2   PREP TIME: 10 MIN.   COOKING TIME: 15 MIN.

Ingredients

2 tbsp ghee, divided
2 chicken breasts, sliced into 1/2 inch pieces
3 cups Brussels sprouts, halved
1/4 cup slivered almonds
Salt and pepper to taste
1 cup fresh parsley, chopped
1 large apple, chopped

Directions

1. Heat 1 tbsp ghee in a large skillet (cast iron skillet works well) over medium-high heat. Add sliced chicken, salt, and pepper and cook 6-8 minutes, flipping once.

2. Remove chicken from heat and set aside on a plate.

3. Add 1 tbsp ghee to Brussels sprouts, slivered almonds, salt, and pepper. Cook for 10-15 minutes, occasionally turning Brussels sprouts. Add cooked chicken and apple to skillet and cook 1-2 minutes.

4. Remove from heat and top with chopped parsley. Enjoy warm.

CALORIES: 503, CARBOHYDRATE 42 GR, PROTEIN: 35 GR, FAT: 25 GR

SHRIMP ASPARAGUS PASTA

SERVINGS: 2   PREP TIME: 5 MIN.   COOKING TIME: 20-30 MIN.

Ingredients

6 oz dry casava flour pasta of your choice
1 tbsp ghee
1 tbsp chopped garlic
1 cup asparagus(chopped)
1/2 lb shrimp
2 tbsp chopped parsley
Salt and pepper to taste

Directions

1. Cook pasta per the directions on the packaging, strain, and set aside.

2. In a large sauté pan, melt the ghee over medium heat.

3. Once the ghee is hot, add the garlic and sauté for 2-3 minutes.

4. Add the chopped asparagus and shrimp to the sauté pan and cook for 5-7 minutes, or until the shrimp is fully cooked.

5. Stir in the pasta and chopped parsley.

6. Season with salt and pepper to taste. Serve hot and enjoy!

CALORIES: 477, CARBOHYDRATE 70 GR, PROTEIN: 25 GR, FAT: 11 GR

Traditional Steak & Potatoes

SERVINGS: 2 PREP TIME: 5 MIN. COOKING TIME: 45-60 MIN.

Ingredients

12 oz grass-fed ribeye steak
2 tbsp ghee
Salt and pepper
2 small russet potatoes
2 tbsp chopped chives

Directions

1. Preheat the oven to 425 F.

2. Pierce the potatoes with a fork, wrap them in aluminum foil, and place in the oven to bake.

3. Season the ribeye with salt and pepper on both sides and set aside at room temperature.

4. Heat a cast iron skillet to medium-high heat.

5. Add the ghee to the cast iron skillet.

6. Once hot, place the ribeye steak in the cast iron skillet and allow it to sear on one side for 3-4 minutes before flipping (for a medium-rare steak).

7. Once seared on both sides, set aside to cool before slicing.

8. Once the potatoes are cooked (easily pierced with a fork) remove them from the oven.

9. Slice the potato, top with ghee and chives, and serve with the ribeye. Enjoy!

CALORIES: 535, CARBOHYDRATE 39 GR, PROTEIN: 41 GR, FAT: 22 GR

Bonus Content

Hormone Balancing Foods Cheat Sheet

Clean Protein

- Grass fed meats (beef, lamb, buffalo, bison)
- Wild-caught fish (salmon, mackerel, tuna and sardines)
- Pasture-raised chicken and turkey
- Organic eggs
- Organic lentils and beans

Healthy Fats

- Olive oil
- Coconut oil/milk/butter
- Grass-fed ghee or butter (unless sensitive to dairy)
- Animal fats from grass-fed animals
- Avocados
- Nuts and seeds & nut and seed butters
- Organic dairy from cows, goats, or sheep
  (full fat cheese, full fat raw milk, kefir)
- Fish oil and cod liver oil

Organic Fruits

- Berries
- Pomegranate
- Acai
- Apples
- Grapefruit
- Cantaloupe
- Pears
- Figs
- Apricots
- Cherries
- Peaches
- Ripe plantains

Organic Vegetables

- Dark leafy greens
- Broccoli
- Cauliflower
- Brussels sprouts
- Kale
- Beets
- Squash,
- Pumpkin
- Carrots

Resistant Starches

- Sweet potatoes
- Cooked and cooled white potatoes
- Squash
- Organic oats
- Green plantains or under ripe bananas

Gluten-free Grains

- Buckwheat
- Amaranth
- Quinoa
- Rice

Sea Vegetables

- Wakame
- Nori
- Dulse
- Arame
- Agar
- Seaweed salad

Resistant Starches

- Sweet potatoes
- Cooked white potatoes
- Squash
- Organic oats
- Green plantains
- Under ripe bananas

BONUS CONTENT

Nutrient Cheat Sheet
for Menopause and Perimenopause[4]

As you undergo changes to your hormone levels, your body might require certain vitamins more than it used to. These include vitamins that support adrenal function, help balance hormone levels, and aid in improving specific issues that arise from low estrogen levels, such as bone loss.

VITAMIN E

Vitamin E plays an important role in supporting the adrenal glands. These glands are responsible for the synthesis of a small percentage of the body's total estrogen levels. Therefore, they become particularly important during menopause. If the adrenal glands are functioning properly, then when the ovaries stop producing estrogen, the glands will still be producing and releasing some estrogen into the bloodstream. This slight increase in estrogen levels can help relieve some of the symptoms of

---

[4] The information provided is for educational purposes only and does not take the place of medical advice. Talk to your doctor before taking supplements.

menopause. Research has shown that vitamin E supplementation during menopause helps ease symptoms such as hot flashes and night sweats. Sunflower seeds, avocados, almonds, Swiss chard, and butternut squash are all rich in vitamin E.

THE B VITAMINS

The B vitamins (especially vitamin B5) have several functions in the body, including regulating and supporting the adrenal glands. Vitamin B5 (also known as pantothenic acid) is especially important in the production and metabolism of hormones synthesized by the adrenal glands. It plays a role in the synthesis of cholesterol, which is the precursor to all the steroid hormones (including estrogen and progesterone). The B vitamins are heavily involved in energy production and help with memory, regulation of mood, and cognitive functioning. This group of vitamins can minimize "brain fog," which is the difficulty concentrating and poor memory that some women experience in menopause. Vitamin B5 is found in chicken, oats, whole grains, eggs, beef, and potatoes.

VITAMIN C

Vitamin C provides adrenal support, but it also functions in a lot of other pathways that work hard to keep us healthy. It is an important player in the immune system and bone health as well. The adrenal glands are concentrated with vitamin C and use this nutrient to synthesize cortisol, the stress hormone. However, suppose the adrenal glands become overworked and fatigued (which happens when we're under a lot of stress). In that case, the supply of vitamin C might run low. A diet rich in vitamin C ensures that you provide your adrenal glands with enough of this vitamin to function properly and keep the hormones balanced, even when they're under stress. Vitamin C also provides a protective factor against bone loss because it is an important nutrient in the synthesis of collagen. Collagen is the abundant protein in our bones and connective tissues that makes them durable and strong. Adequate intake of vitamin C is easily obtained through diet alone. Citrus fruits, such as lemons and oranges, grapefruits, red peppers, and Brussels sprouts all contain a very high percentage of your daily recommended intake of vitamin C. One orange already contains over 100 percent of the vitamin C that you need!

CALCIUM

Almost all of the calcium in our bodies is found in the skeletal system (over 99 percent). It is the main mineral component of bone. When estrogen levels decrease in menopause, the risks of osteoporosis significantly increase. Estrogen has protective effects against osteoporosis and bone loss. Thus, calcium is essential during this stage in your life because you must ensure that your bones get enough of the required nutrients to stay as strong and healthy as possible, even with lower estrogen levels. Dairy products (such as organic kefir and full-fat yogurt) are known for being rich in calcium, but sardines, nuts, and seeds are also excellent sources of this mineral. You should also make sure you're getting an adequate intake of vitamin D, which many individuals are deficient in. Vitamin D is essential for the effective absorption of calcium.

SUPERFOODS FOR PERIMENOPAUSE MENOPAUSE

POMEGRANATE

Pomegranate contains estrogen-like compounds that are structurally like the female estrogen estrone. Pomegranate contains the highest amount of steroidal estrogens compared to any other plant-based source. Pomegranate also helps modulate estrogen and act as an aromatase inhibitor. While you can eat pomegranates, experts suggest pomegranate extract or pomegranate seed oil.

LIGAN RICH SEEDS, GRAINS, AND LEGUMES

Four main plant constituent groups have demonstrated weak estrogenic activity; however only lignans and isoflavones have shown specific human estrogenic activity. You get lignans from seeds, whole grains, legumes, vegetables, and some fruits. Because lignans are abundant in grains and legumes, I do not recommend a Paleo diet for menopausal women. However, I suggest you soak, sprout, or ferment your grains and legumes to make them more digestible.

ISOFLAVONE RICH SOYBEANS

Soy is also well-known for its estrogenic effects. Some studies have found that women who were in menopause and who ate a diet rich in soy had improvements to their joints and bone health, something that deteriorates following the decrease in estrogen. Soy might also reduce the common symptoms of menopause, including hot flashes, excessive sweating, and heart palpitations, which can sometimes occur. It is the Isoflavones in soy that provide the estrogenic effects. Safe sources of soy are sprouted organic tofu, organic soybeans, organic miso, and organic soymilk. It's essential to purchase non-GMO and organic soy only.

PORTOBELLO MUSHROOMS

Portobello mushrooms are good source of vitamin D and B12 that we need as we age. Other mushrooms, too, such as cordyceps and reishi, have estrogen-modulating effects and may help reduce common menopause symptoms.

PROTEIN POWDERS

Blood sugar stability is essential for hormone balance. Unfortunately, many of the protein powders on the market have ingredients that may inhibit hormones. Avoid highly processed protein powders with isolates such as soy, whey, and grain-based powders. Look for hemp, pumpkin, chicken, beef, or bone broth protein powder. I suggest Nutiva, Sunwarrior, Vital Proteins, Ancient Nutrition, or Rootcology protein powders. If these are out of your budget, don't compromise on quality. It would be better to pass than bring in poor-quality proteins that may inhibit hormone balance.

PROBIOTICS

Cultured foods help keep the gut microbiome thriving. Research is emerging, demonstrating a connection between the gut microbiome and hormone health. Researchers now believe that certain microbes in the gut secrete and modulate hormones to such an extent that the gut microbiota should be classified as part of the endocrine system! To cultivate a robust gut microbiome, you should incorporate cultured foods such as cultured vegetables, sauerkraut, beet kvass, sugar-free non-dairy yogurt, and kefir waters.

ORGANIC PASTURE-RAISED EGGS

Studies show eggs boost testosterone! Organic eggs are filled with even more important nutrients than conventional eggs – especially omega-3 fats. Conventional eggs also have soy. a by-product in most chicken feeds.

In general, eggs are a cheaper source of protein and healthy fats than meat, so buying organic is worth a little more. Eggs are a complete protein source, meaning they contain every essential amino acid you need. They contain omega-3 fatty acids, vitamins A and E, beta-carotene, and choline, which is important for fetal brain development.

SHATAVARI

Shatavari is wild asparagus. In Ayurveda, it is considered a female tonic. Traditionally it has been used to boost libido, tame hot flashes, curb night sweating, and lessen brain fog. Shatavari also has immunomodulating, apoptogenic, and anti-stress effects.

Customarily shatavari is mixed with a glass of warm milk and honey. Still, it can be incorporated into various dishes, drinks, and teas. You can purchase shatavari powder on Amazon.

BONUS CONTENT

Your Hormone-Hacking Weight-loss Checklist

Top 10 Goals *(Specific, Measurable, Achievable)*

1. My Specific Goals

> *EX: Lose 10 pounds over the next 12 weeks.*
> *Improve my energy levels and overall well-being.*

Timeline

> *I aim to achieve my weight-loss goals over the next three months.*

Reasons for Wanting to Lose Weight

> *EX: To feel more confident, improve health, and*
> *reduce stress on my joints*

2. Stress-Management Techniques
Meditation

EX: I will practice 10 minutes of mindfulness meditation each morning

Deep Breathing Exercises

EX: Whenever I feel stressed, I will practice deep breathing techniques for a few minutes.

3. Food Journal

Date

Food Intake

Breakfast

Lunch

Snack

Dinner

Emotions

Date

Food Intake

Breakfast

Lunch

Snack

Dinner

Emotions

Date
Food Intake
Breakfast
Lunch
Snack
Dinner
Emotions

Date
Food Intake
Breakfast
Lunch
Snack
Dinner
Emotions

Date
Food Intake
Breakfast
Lunch
Snack
Dinner
Emotions

4. Balanced Meal Planning

Breakfast

EX: Protein smoothies with spinach, almond milk, protein powder, and nut butter

Lunch

EX: Quinoa bowl with roasted vegetables, chickpeas, and tahini dressing.

Dinner

EX: Grilled lean meats (chicken, turkey) with a side of sautéed leafy greens.

5. Hormonal Health

Hormone-Supporting Foods & Nutrients

EX: Omega-3 fatty acids from fatty fish, flax seeds, and chia seeds. Cruciferous vegetables like broccoli and cauliflower support estrogen metabolism. Probiotic-rich foods like yogurt and fermented foods promote gut health.

6. Physical Activity

Exercise Routine

Cardio

30 minutes of brisk walking or cycling five days a week

Strength Training

Full-body strength training exercises twice a week.

Stretching

Full-body strength training exercises twice a week.

7. Sleep Optimization

Sleep Routine

EX: Aim for 7-8 hours of sleep each night. Create a relaxing bedtime routine, such as reading a book or taking a warm bath before bed.

8. Hydration

Daily Water Intake Goal

Drink at least half your body weight in ounces of water per day

Ways to Stay Hydrated

Carry a reusable water bottle throughout the day and set reminders to drink water.

9. Social Support

EX: I joined a local yoga class, where I met some friendly people with similar health goals. I also connected with an online community of women focusing on hormonal health and weight management.

10. Track Progress

Weight-loss Progress

EX: Starting weight - 175 lbs, Current weight - 170 lbs.

Non-scale Victories

EX: I noticed that my energy levels have improved, and I feel more positive overall.

Super Savvy Tip

Download your FREE copy of
my beautiful, full-color
Hormone-Hacking for Weight-loss Checklist:

hackyourhormonesforweightloss.com/bonuses

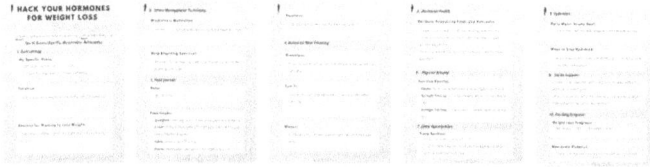